50 KETO DIET RECIPES

Simple and Delicious Ketogenic Diet Recipes Book - 50 Recipes for a Healthy Life.

JENNY BROOKS

TABLE OF CONTENTS

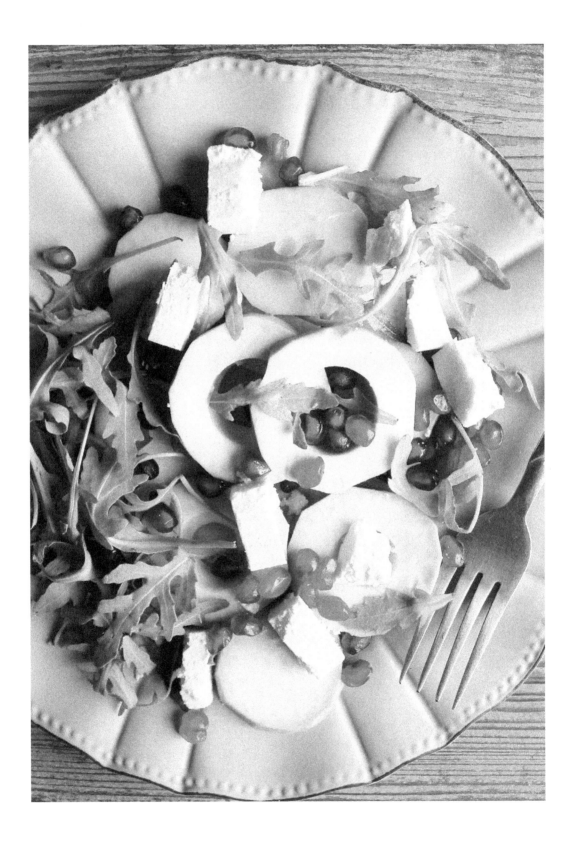

LOW CARB OLIVE GARDEN ZUPPA TOSCANA

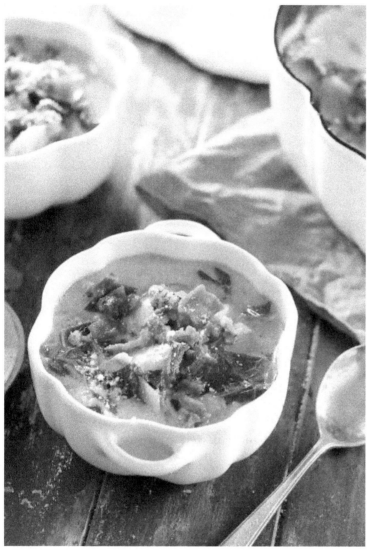

A delicious copycat recipe that uses turnips instead of potatoes!

SERVINGS: 6

INGREDIENTS:

5 small turnips

3 kale leaves

1 onion

4 cloves garlic

190 g bacon slices (around 6 slices)

1500 ml chicken broth

250 ml heavy cream (almond milk for paleo)

1 tsp salt

5 Tbsp parmesan Homemade Italian Sausage

200 g ground chicken

200 g ground pork

2 tsp sage

½ tsp garlic powder

½ tsp salt

½ tsp black pepper

½ tsp chili flakes

¼ tsp cayenne pepper (optional)

½ tsp paprika

DIRECTIONS:

01. Peel and dice the turnips. Chop the kale into bite-size pieces. Dice the onion. Mince the garlic. Slice the bacon into 1cm slices.

02. In a bowl, add the sausage ingredients and mix well with your hands.

03. In a large pot, cook the bacon rashes on medium heat until nice and crispy. Do not drain the excess oil. Transfer the bacon to the side.

04. In the same pot, add the sausage and cook until browned, 3-5 minutes. Set aside. Again, do not drain the leftover oil.

05. Add the chopped onion and garlic to the pot and cook for 3-4 minutes until tender. Add the chicken broth and turnips. Turn the heat to high and put to boil for about 5-7 minutes. The turnips will soften very quickly. Pierce with a fork to check from time to time.

06. Once the turnips are soft, turn the heat down, add the kale and cook until wilted, around a minute. Add the heavy cream, salt and stir. Add the cooked sausages to the pot and stir.

07. The soup is now done. If you think it's not salty enough, just add a bit more.

08. Serve and sprinkle the crispy bacon and parmesan over each serving bowl.

NUTRITION:

Calories 459

Calories from Fat 321

Total Fat 35.68 g

Saturated Fat 13.91 g

Polyunsaturated Fat 3.17 g

Monounsaturated Fat 13.09 g

Cholesterol 123 mg

Sodium 1472 mg

Potassium 514 mg

Total Carbohydrates 12.36 g

Dietary Fiber 2.3 g

Sugars 4.57 g

Protein 22.25 g

PARMESAN WINGS

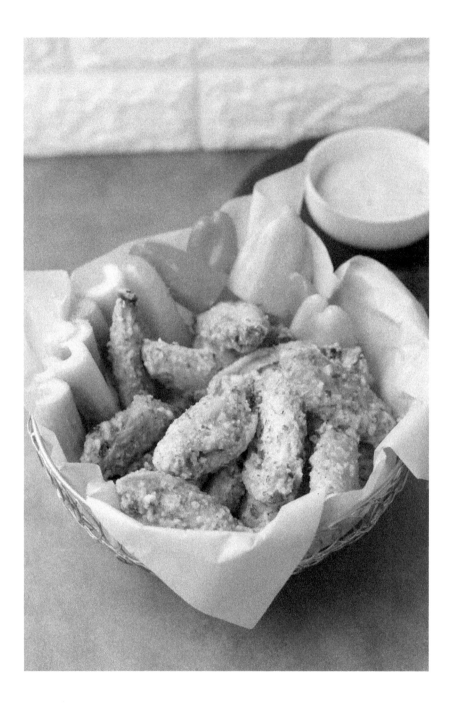

SERVINGS: 6

INGREDIENTS:

2 lb chicken wings, thawed if frozen

1 tsp sea salt

2 Tbsp baking powder

½ cup salted butter, melted

½ cup grated Parmesan cheese

1 clove garlic, minced

1 Tbsp chopped fresh flat-leaf parsley

1 ½ tsp garlic powder

½ tsp onion powder

¼ tsp ground black pepper

NUTRITION:

Calories 468

Fat 38 g

Carbohydrates 2 g

Fiber 0 g

Protein 30 g

DIRECTIONS:

01. Spread the wings in a single layer across some paper towels and sprinkle with the salt. Cover with another layer of paper towels and let rest for 20 minutes.

02. Place an oven rack in the middle-lower position and another rack in the middle upper position. Preheat the oven to 250°F. Set a cooling rack on a rimmed baking sheet.

03. Combine the wings and baking powder in a resalable plastic bag. Shake to coat the wings evenly.

04. Spread the wings in a single layer across the cooling rack. Bake on the middle-lower oven rack for 30 minutes.

05. Increase the oven temperature to 425°F and move the baking sheet to the middle-upper rack. Bake the wings for an additional 45 minutes, or until the skin is nice and crispy.

06. While the wings are baking, make the sauce: Combine the melted butter, Parmesan cheese, minced garlic, parsley, garlic powder, onion powder, and pepper in a medium bowl.

07. Remove the wings from the oven and let rest for 5 minutes. Toss in the sauce before serving.

BLT STUFFED AVOCADO

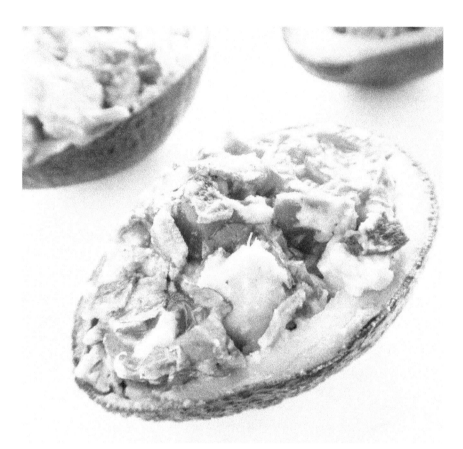

This BLT stuffed avocado recipe makes a perfect lunch or snack. It's naturally healthy, low carb, paleo, and gluten-free

SERVINGS: 4

INGREDIENTS:

2 medium Avocado

2 slices Bacon

½ cup Grape tomatoes (halved)

½ cup Romaine lettuce (chopped)

1 tsp Lime juice

¼ tsp Garlic powder

¼ tsp Sea salt

⅛ Tsp Black pepper

DIRECTIONS:

01. Place bacon onto a skillet while the skillet is still cold. Cook the bacon over low or medium-low heat until the edges start to curl. Flip and continue cooking until golden and crispy. This process may take 5 minutes or maybe a little longer. Drain on paper towels (it will crisp up more as it cools).

02. Meanwhile, slice the avocados in half and remove the pits. Scoop half of the flesh out of each avocado half (leave half undisturbed) and transfer to a bowl.

03. Mash the avocado in the bowl. Stir in the grape tomatoes, lettuce, lime juice, garlic powder, sea salt, and black pepper (adjust seasonings to taste if needed).

NUTRITION:

Calories 189

Fat 16 g

Protein 4 g

Total Carbs 10 g

Net Carbs 3 g

Fiber 7 g

Sugar 1 g

EASY BUFFALO CHICKEN DIP

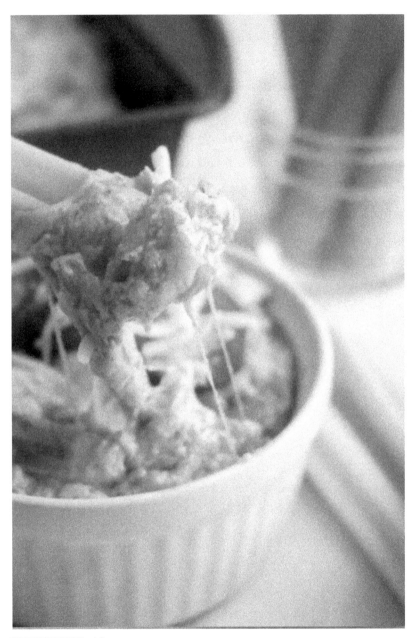

SERVINGS: 10

INGREDIENTS:

3 cups shredded chicken (cooked) we used a rotisserie chicken

¾ cup Blue Cheese Dressing

¾ cup Franks Red Hot Sauce

12 oz Cream Cheese

1 cup shredded mozzarella cheese

¼ cup jalapenos (optional, for topping)

DIRECTIONS:

01. Add cream cheese and hot sauce to a medium heat saucepan.

02. Once fully combined stir in the blue cheese dressing and chicken.

03. Once fully incorporated, slowly mix in 3/4 cup of the mozzarella cheese.

04. Once fully incorporated transfer mixture to an 8x8 baking dish. Layer the rest of the mozzarella cheese on top.

05. Place in a 350 degree oven for 15 minutes.

06. Serve warm and enjoy!

NUTRITION:

Calories 346.5 kcal

Carbohydrates 2.4 g

Protein 20 g

Fat 28 g

Net Carbs 2.4 g

CHICKEN LETTUCE WRAPS

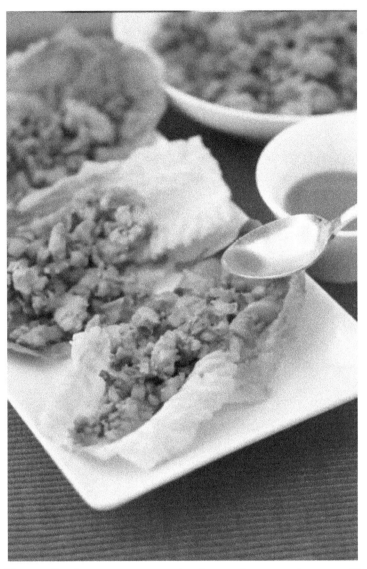

For a dipping sauce, we mixed together equal parts dijon mustard and coconut aminos/tamari. You can also add a little chili oil or Sriracha if you like it hot!

INGREDIENTS:

For The Filling:

1 lb ground chicken (we ground raw chicken thighs or chicken breast in our food processor)

6–8 oz button or baby bella mushrooms, finely minced

1 (8oz) can water chestnuts, drained and minced

2 green onions, sliced 2 tsp fresh ginger, minced 1 clove garlic, minced

1 Tbsp avocado oil (olive or coconut oil would work well too)

¼–1/3 cup coconut aminos, GF tamari, or soy sauce

To Serve:

Lettuce leaves (romaine hearts or iceberg lettuce work well) Cilantro

DIRECTIONS:

01. Prepare the filling by heating the oil in a medium sauté pan over medium heat. Add chicken and cook until lightly browned and cooked all the way through.

02. Add mushrooms, water chestnuts, green onions, ginger, and garlic. Cook until fragrant and cooked through. Add 4 Tbsp coconut aminos or tamari and stir to coat chicken mixture.

03. Add additional sauce as desired (remember you don't want it too wet, or it will make eating your lettuce wraps a very messy, soggy experience).

04. Scoop mixture onto lettuce leaves. top with cilantro, if desired, and your favorite dipping sauce.

NUTRITION:

Calories Per Serving 230

Total Fat 6.9 g

Cholesterol 82.7 mg

Sodium 638.3 mg

Total Carbohydrate 12.5 g

Dietary Fiber 3 g

Sugars 3.9 g

Protein 29.9 g

ANTIPASTO SKEWERS

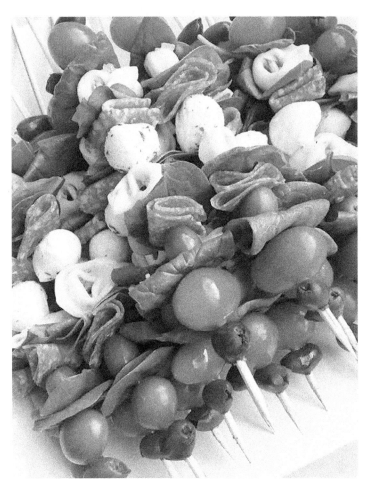

These antipasto skewers are quick to make. They are perfect for any dinner party or an easy New Year's Eve appetizer recipe!

SERVINGS: 16

INGREDIENTS:

8 Prosciutto, slices

16 Ciliegine, (1 inch) mozzarella balls

16 Sun dried tomatoes, , in oil

16 Basil leaves

DIRECTIONS:

01. Cut prosciutto slices in half.

02. Fold up prosciutto and place one sun dried tomato, one basil leaf, and one mozzarella ball on top of it.

03. Skewer with a toothpick.

NUTRITION:

Calories per Serving 230

Total Fat 6.9 g

Cholesterol 82.7 mg

Sodium 638.3 mg

Total Carbohydrate 12.5 g

Dietary Fiber 3 g

Sugars 3.9 g

Protein 29.9 g

LOW-CARB TORTILLA CHIPS

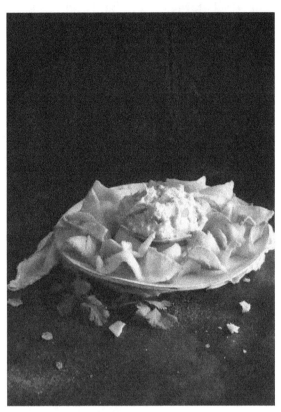

This recipe for the Best Low-Carb Tortilla Chips makes a perfect snack for dipping. Best of all, these chips work for low-carb, Atkins, ketogenic, lc/hf, gluten-free, grain free, and Banting diets.

SERVINGS: 6

INGREDIENTS:

2 cups part-skim grated mozzarella cheese

¾ cup super fine almond flour

½ tsp salt

Optional: ½ teaspoon chili powder

NUTRITION:

Amount   Per   1/4 recipe

Calories 280

Fat 23 g

Carbs 7 g

Fiber 2 g

Protein 21 g

Net Carbs 5 g

DIRECTIONS:

01. Preheat oven to 375° F. Cut 2 pieces of parchment about 20 inches long. Have a rolling pin and 2 cookie sheets available.

02. Prepare a double boiler. A pot partially filled with water with a mixing bowl that fits on top works well for this purpose. Over high heat, bring the water in the pot to a simmer, then turn heat to low.

03. In the bowl part of the double boiler, add the cheese, almond flour, chili powder (if using), and salt. Using caution to not to get burned by the steam, place the bowl over the pot of simmering water. I use a silicone mitten to hold the bowl. Stir ingredients constantly.

04. As the cheese melts, the ingredients will start to develop a doughy appearance. When it starts to hold together in a ball, turn it out onto a piece of parchment paper.

05. While the dough is hot, but not hot enough to burn your hands, knead the dough to completely mix the ingredients.

06. Divide the dough into 2 equal sections.

07. Form one section into a ball and place on a piece of parchment paper. Pat into a rectangular shape, then cover with another piece of parchment. Using the rolling pin, roll into about a 9 inch by 15 inch rectangle. Dough should be fairly thin. You may need to turn the dough and straighten the parchment if it wrinkles. Remove the top piece of parchment and place the bottom piece of parchment containing the dough non a cutting board. Using a pizza cutter, cut dough into squares or triangles. Slide the parchment with the triangles onto the cookie sheet. Arrange the triangles of dough so they are at least 1/2 inch away from each other. Set aside.

08. Repeat for the second ball of dough.

09. Place the cookie sheets with the tortilla chips in the oven. Bake for 5-8 minutes or until the centers turn golden brown. Watch them carefully as it is easy to burn them.

10. Remove them from oven and slide them onto a cooling rack using a spatula.

11. Chips will become crunchier as they cool.

KETO PIGS IN A BLANKET

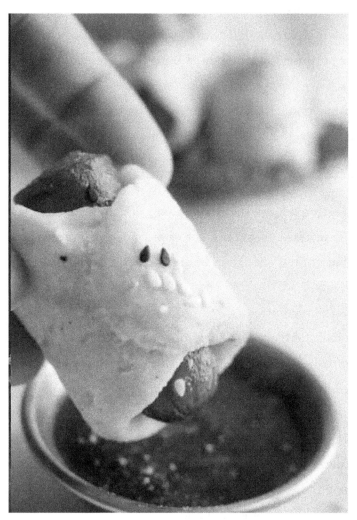

SERVINGS: 4

INGREDIENTS:

4 medium hot dogs

½ cup Shredded mozzarella cheese

¾ cup Almond Flour

1 large Egg

¼ tsp Baking powder

¼ tsp garlic powder

½ tsp Pink Himalayan Salt

½ tsp Sesame Seeds

DIRECTIONS:

01. Cut each hot dog into 3 equal sized pieces and set aside.

02. Melt mozzarella in microwave and add almond flour and egg. Combine well.

03. Add baking powder, garlic and salt. Combine well.

04. Form dough in hands and split into 12 equal sized pieces and roll into dough.

05. Place dough balls onto a parchment lined baking sheet. Press each ball into oval shape.

06. Place each hot dog piece into the dough and wrap like a blanket.

07. Sprinkle with sesame seeds (press down so they stick to dough).

08. Place pigs in 350 degree oven for 17-20 minutes.

09. Serve warm and enjoy!

NUTRITION:

Calories 332.25 kcal

Carbohydrates 7.25 g

Protein 16.25 g

Fat 27.5 g

Fiber 2.25 g

SUGAR-FREE GRANOLA BARS

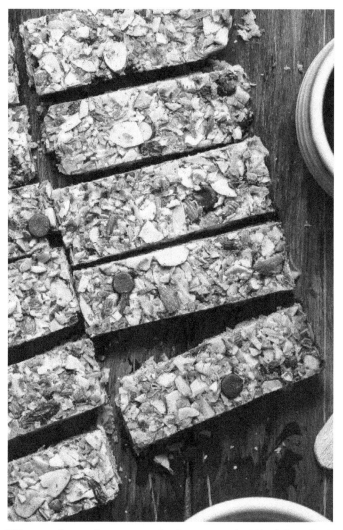

Want to know how to make homemade Kind Bars? Try this Kind Bar recipe copycat. They're the easiest low carb, gluten-free, sugar-free granola bars ever.

SERVINGS: 12

INGREDIENTS:

2 cups Almonds

* ½ cup Pumpkin seeds *

 1/3 cup Coconut flakes (unsweetened)

2 Tbsp Hemp seeds

¼ cup Sukrin Fiber Syrup Clear

¼ cup Almond butter

¼ cup Powdered erythritol (or any powdered sweetener)

2 tsp Vanilla extract ½ tsp Sea salt (omit if almonds and pumpkin seeds are salted)

2 medium Vanilla bean

DIRECTIONS:

01. Line an 8x8 in (20x20 cm) baking pan with parchment paper.

02. In a large bowl, stir together the almonds, pumpkin seeds, coconut flakes, and hemp seeds. Set aside.

03. In a large saucepan, heat the fiber syrup, almond butter, powdered erythritol and sea salt for a couple of minutes, until easy to stir. Stir until smooth.

04. Remove from heat. Stir in the vanilla extract and vanilla bean seeds.

05. Stir the syrup mixture into the nut mixture.

06. Transfer the mixture to a lined baking dish and press firmly to create a smooth top. Use a large, flat spatula to create an even flat surface and press down firmly.

07. Cool completely on the counter. When fully cooled, gently lift the parchment out of the pan and transfer on top of a cutting board. Use a sharp chef's knife to cut into bars using a firm downward motion (don't see-saw back and forth).

NUTRITION:

Calories 216

Fat 18 g

Protein 8 g

Total Carbs 7 g

Net Carbs 3 g

Fiber 4 g

Sugar 1 g

LOW CARB ONION RINGS

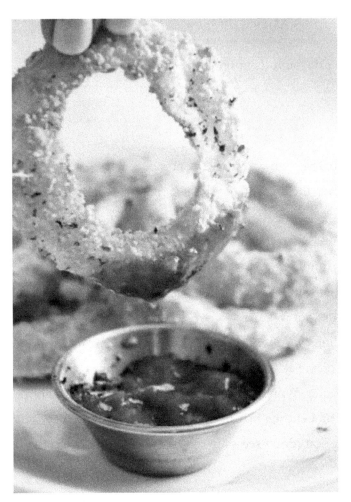

SERVINGS: 2

INGREDIENTS:

1 medium white onion

½ cup Coconut flour

2 large eggs

1 Tbsp Heavy Whipping Cream

2 oz Pork Rinds

½ cup grated parmesan cheese

DIRECTIONS:

01. Slice onion width wise in half inch thick rings.

02. Break apart rings and set aside all the inside pieces you won't be using.

03. Use three different bowls to make a coconut flour, egg wash and heavy whipping cream, and pork rind parmesan coating stations.

04. Starting with coconut flour go through all the steps of coating and place on baking rack as pictured above.

05. Once all onions are coated, double back and recoat them starting with the egg wash.

06. TIP: reprocess or remake the pork rind parmesan coating if it begins soggy/clumpy.

07. Places double coated rings back on greased baking rack and place in 425 degree oven for 15 minutes.

08. Serve warm and enjoy!

NUTRITION:

Calories 211 kcal

Carbohydrates 7.5 g

Protein 16 g

Fat 12.5 g

Fiber 3 g

Net Carbs 4.5 g

LOW CARB BLUEBERRY MUFFINS

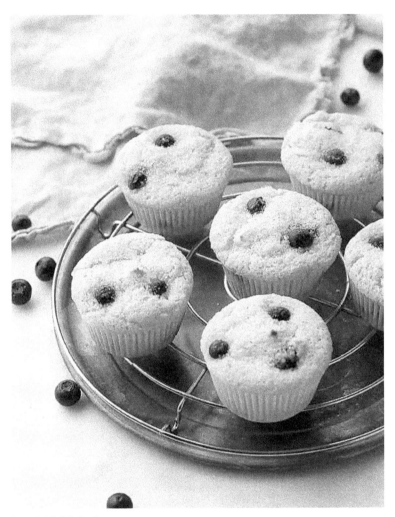

SERVINGS: 6

INGREDIENTS:

Cream Together

½ stick (2 oz) butter, very soft

4 Tbsp (2 oz) cream cheese, very soft

½ tsp vanilla

Dry INGREDIENTS:

½ cup coconut flour

¼ cup Swerve Granulated

1 tsp baking powder

¼ tsp salt

1/16 tsp cinnamon

1/8 tsp xanthan gum (binds ingredients)

Wet ingredients

3 large eggs (cold)

¼ cup heavy cream (last wet addition)

Add Last

1/3 cup fresh blueberries

2 tsp Swerve Granulated

DIRECTIONS:

Preheat oven to 350°. Position oven rack to the lower third of the oven. Line a six cup muffin tin with paper liners. Add the dry ingredients together in a smaller bowl and whisk together to combine and break up any lumps.

Combine:

01. In a medium bowl, cream the butter, cream cheese, and vanilla together until light and fluffy. Add 1 egg and beat into the butter mixture until the mixture is light and fluffy (it may break or separate, it's okay). Add 1/3 of the dry ingredients and mix until completely incorporated, making sure to keep that light, fluffy texture. Keep in mind that we want a light and fluffy — almost mousse-like texture throughout this process.
02. Add another egg and beat until fully combined and the batter is fluffy. Add half of the remaining dry ingredients, beating again. Add the last egg, beating until fully incorporated, followed by the last of the dry ingredients. Finish by adding the heavy cream, once again, beating until the batter is thick, but still light and fluffy. Fold in the blueberries.

Filling the Muffin Tin:

01. Spoon the thick batter into a plastic zip-loc bag and snip off a corner, producing about a 3/4 inch hole. Place the snipped corner into a muffin liner and squeeze the batter into a fat, rounded mound, filling the muffin liner about 3/4 full. Repeat for each muffin liner, adding any remaining batter to those that need a little more. Knock down any peaks with your finger. Sprinkle about ¼ teaspoon of Swerve granulated over the top of each muffin to help prevent burning and to give the muffins a nice look.

Bake: 01. Place the muffins into the oven. Turn the oven up to 400° degrees for 5 minutes. Then, turn the oven back to 350° and bake the blueberry muffins for about 25 minutes more. They're ready when they feel firm when lightly pressed with a finger, but still sound a little moist. Remove from the oven and let cool five minutes before gently removing from the pan and placing on a cooling rack.

NUTRITION:

Calories 273

Fat 25 g

Protein 5 g

Total Carbs 7 g

Fiber 3 g

Net Carbs 4 g

KALE CHIPS

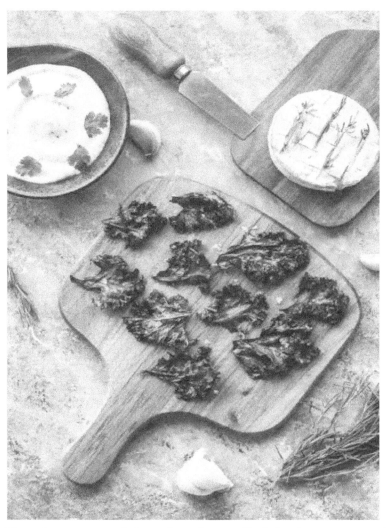

If you have never tried putting pieces of kale in the oven to make kale chips, then this is going to be your new favorite recipe. The crunch from these crispy baked leaves is just insatiable. Paired with some baked camembert, onion dip, and some salami crackers, you've got yourself a mega snack board suitable for anyone on a ketogenic diet.

INGREDIENTS:

1 Bunch Kale

2 Tbsp olive oil

½ tsp Salt

½ tsp Italian Herbs (oregano)

DIRECTIONS:

01. Preheat your oven to 180C (355F)

02. Separate each large leaf out from the bunch of kale. Pat them down dry so that you don't need to bake out any extra moisture

03. Remove the large stalk from the middle of the kale leaf, and then slice the remaining kale into large chunk as shown in the picture.

04. Place the large chunks into a large mixing bowl, and cover with olive oil. Make sure you mix them around to get a good coverage all over

05. In a large baking pan, place some baking paper over the pan and put as many pieces of kale as you can fit. Sprinkle with salt and a little Italian herbs

06. Place them into the oven for 10 mins, or until crispy. (Depending on the quality of the kale, you might have to cook for a little longer)

NUTRITION:

Calories 74

Calories from Fat 63

Total Fat 7 g

Saturated Fat 1 g

Polyunsaturated Fat 1 g

Monounsaturated Fat 5 g

Sodium 250 mg

Potassium 122 mg

Total Carbohydrates 3g

Dietary Fiber 1 g

Sugars 0.02 g

Protein 1 g

PORTOBELLO MUSHROOM MINI KETO PIZZA

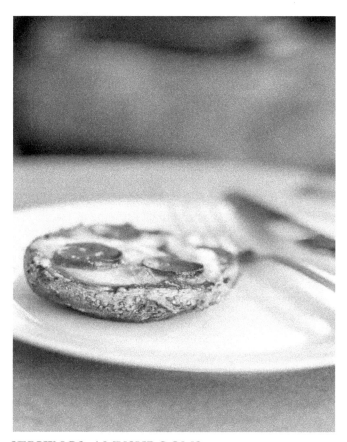

SERVINGS: 4 MUSHROOMS

INGREDIENTS:

4 Large Portobello Mushrooms

100 g Low carb marinara sauce (½ Cup)

80 g fresh or grated mozzarella

20 slices pepperoni or chorizo sausage

DIRECTIONS:

01. (Optional First Step) — Arrange mushrooms onto ovenproof tray, gills up. Sprinkle with salt and cook in oven heated to 375°F (190°C) for 20 minutes. Remove from oven and drain away liquid from pan and mushrooms.

02. Arrange mushrooms onto baking tray, gill up. Spread 2 tbsp marinara sauce onto each, followed by 1/4 of the mozzarella (approx 20g or 2 tbsp). Finally arrange 5 slices of pepperoni onto each pizza

03. Bake in the over for 20 minutes at 375°F (190°C) until cheese begins to turn golden and bubbly. Serve immediately.

NUTRITION:

Amount Per Mushroom Pizza

Net Carbs 4 g

Fats 9 g

Protein 8 g

KETO POPCORN RECIPE CHEESE PUFFS

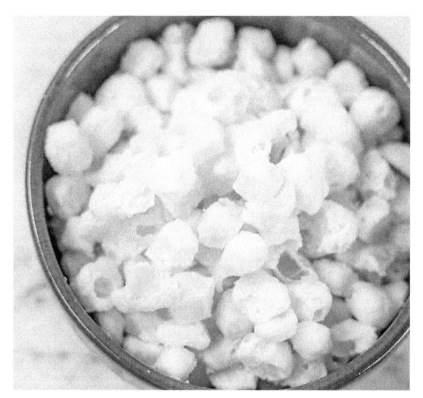

You can buy them but they're much cheaper to make and you can make a bucket load of Keto Popcorn if you like the cheese puffs nicely once dry SERVINGS: 4

INGREDIENTS:

4 oz cheddar cheese sliced

DIRECTIONS:

01. Cut the cheese into small ¼ inch squares.

02. Before baking, this recipe must be prepared 24 hrs beforehand

03. Place on a cookie sheet lined with parchment paper and cover with a clean tea towel (dish towel).

04. Leave the cheese to dry out for at least 24 hours (you might need to leave it longer if it is humid where you live).

05. The next day preheat your oven to 200C/390F and bake the cheese for 3-5

minutes until it is puffed up. 06. Leave to cool for 10 minutes before enjoying

NUTRITION:

Serving 60 g

Calories 114 kcal

Carbohydrates 0 g

Protein 7 g

Fat 9 g

Saturated Fat 5 g

Cholesterol 29 mg

Sodium 176 mg

Potassium 27 mg

Fiber 0 g

Sugar 0 g

KETO TORTILLA CHIPS

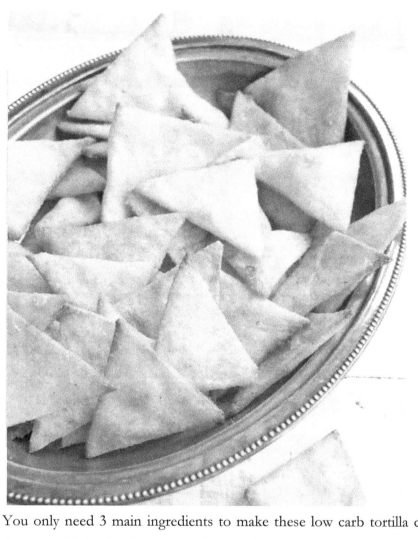

You only need 3 main ingredients to make these low carb tortilla chips. If you roll them out thinly, they become really crunchy.

SERVINGS: 8

INGREDIENTS:

200 g / 2 cups pre-shredded mozzarella

75 g / ¾ cup almond flour ground almonds work well too

2 Tbsp psyllium husk or 2 tsp psyllium husk powder

Pinch salt

Optional: ¼ tsp each garlic powder/onion powder/paprika

DIRECTIONS:

01. Heat your oven to 180 Celsius / 356 Fahrenheit.

02. Melt the mozzarella in the microwave (ca 90 sec-2 min). Alternatively, heat gently in a non-stick pot.

03. Add the almond flour/ground almonds and psyllium husk plus the salt and spices, if using. Stir until combined, then knead until you have a smooth dough.

04. Separate the dough into 2 balls and roll out between 2 sheets of baking/parchment paper. Roll out as thinly as possible! The thinner, the crispier your tortilla chips will turn out.

05. Cut into triangles (I used a pizza cutter) and spread out on a sheet of baking paper so the tortilla chips don't touch.

06. Bake 6-8 minutes or until browned on the edges. Baking time will depend on the thickness of your tortilla chips. I baked mine in 2 rounds, plus a third round for the off-cuts.

NUTRITION:

Calories 143

Calories from Fat 83

Total Fat 9.2 g

Total Carbohydrates 4.8 g

Dietary Fiber 2.9 g

Sugars 0.6 g

Protein 8.3 g

KETO COOKIE DOUGH

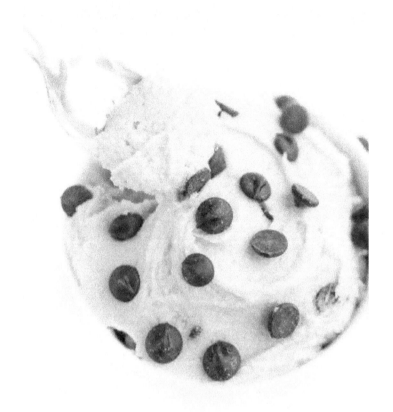

Keto Cookie Dough Recipe for those late night cookie dough cravings. This low carb cookie dough will hit the spot at just 1 Net Carb per serving!

SERVING: 32

INGREDIENTS:

½ cup butter softened (may use coconut butter for dairy-free alternative)

¼ -½ cup erythritol (or powdered erythritol works also)

1/8 tsp liquid stevia optional for extra sweetness

1 tsp vanilla extract

½ tsp sea salt

½ cup heavy cream or coconut milk for dairy-free alternative

¾ cup coconut flour

¼ cup low carb chocolate chips

DIRECTIONS:

01. In a large bowl cream together butter, powdered erythritol, stevia, vanilla extract, salt and heavy cream.

02. Blend in coconut flour and beat together until well combined.

03. 3. Fold in chocolate chips. Eat with a spoon or scoop into bite size pieces as they will become more stiff after refrigerated. Store in the refrigerator.

NUTRITION:

Calories 57

Calories from Fat 45

Total Fat 5 g

Saturated Fat 3 g

Cholesterol 12 mg

Sodium 69 mg

Potassium 2 mg

Total Carbohydrates 3 g

Dietary Fiber 1 g

Sugars 0 g

Protein 0 g

CHEWY KETO CHOCOLATE-CHIP COOKIES

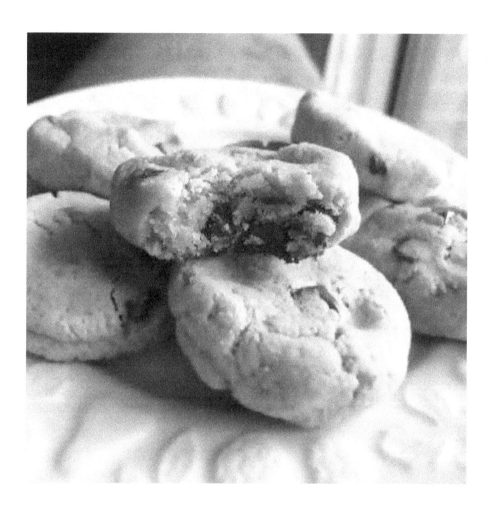

INGREDIENTS:

1 cup (112g) almond flour

¼ cup coconut flour

1 Tbsp (10g) vital wheat gluten OR ¼ tsp xanthan gum

½ tsp baking soda

¼ tsp baking powder

¼ tsp salt

¼ cup + 2 Tbsp (90g) unsalted, room temperature butter

6 ½ Tbsp splenda (OR another sweetener that measures like sugar)

3 ½ Tbsp truvia (OR 6 Tbsp of a sweetener that measures like sugar)

½ tsp blackstrap molasses (optional-adds brown sugar flavour)

1 tsp vanilla extract

2 eggs ¼ cup (60g) stevia-sweetened chocolate-chips

DIRECTIONS:

01. Pre-heat your oven to 350*F.

02. In a large bowl, combine your flours, vital wheat gluten(or xanthan gum), baking soda, baking powder and salt.

03. In another bowl, beat together your butter, sweeteners, vanilla extract and molasses until light and fluffy.

04. Add your eggs and beat again until combined.

05. Pour your wet mixture into the dry and stir to until a thick dough forms.

06. Fold in your chocolate-chips and then place the dough in the refrigerator for 1520min.

07. Spray/grease a baking sheet with oil.

08. Begin rolling your dough into balls (I ended up with 15) and space them evenly apart on the baking sheet.

09. Flatten each one slightly with the back of a spoon and place in the oven.

10. Bake for 8-9min or until the cookies are JUST set and the bottoms lightly browned. (They will continue baking on the cookie sheet afterwards. You can cook longer if you don't like the slightly under-cooked middle…(that's favorite part, haha)).

11. Let the cookies cool on the baking sheet for 15min or so before removing and placing on a plate.

12. Serve immediately or store in an airtight container in the freezer for a quick snack in the future! Enjoy!

NUTRITION:

Fat 11 g

NET Carbs 1.5 g

Protein 4 g

Fiber 3 g

LOW CARB KETO HOT SPINACH AND ARTICHOKE DIP

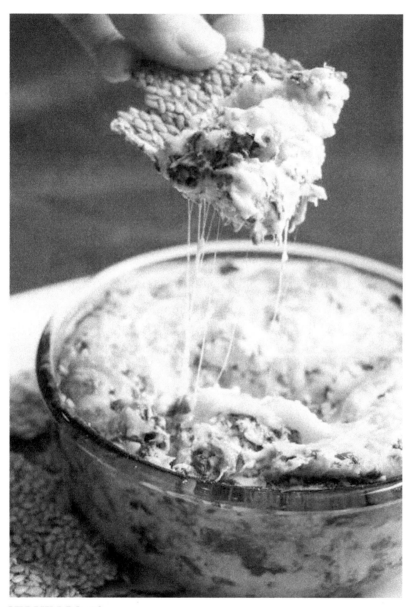

SERVINGS: 10

INGREDIENTS:

4 oz Pancetta diced

8 oz Cream Cheese

8 oz artichoke hearts diced

¼ cup mayo

¼ cup sour cream

½ cup parmesan grated

2 Tbsp garlic powder

½ cup spinach frozen

DIRECTIONS:

01. In a skillet over medium heat, add the diced pancetta and cook until golden brown, roughly 8 minutes.

02. Place another pan over medium heat and add the frozen spinach. Cook until all the water has been cooked out, roughly 8 minutes

03. In the skillet with the browned pancetta, add the cream cheese and lower the heat to medium. Cook until the cream cheese is smooth.

04. Preheat the oven to 350 degrees. In the Skillet with the cream cheese mixture, add in the rest of the ingredients and mix with a spoon until combined.

05. Place in the oven and cook for 15 to 18 minutes. To make the top golden, broil for 3 minutes. Serve with your favorite crackers, pork rinds, vegetables and more.

NUTRITION:

Calories 224

Calories from Fat 180

Total Fat 20 g

Saturated Fat 8 g

Cholesterol 41 mg

Sodium 356 mg

Potassium 93 mg

Total Carbohydrates 3 g

Sugars 1 g

Protein 5 g

KETO PEANUT BUTTER CUPS

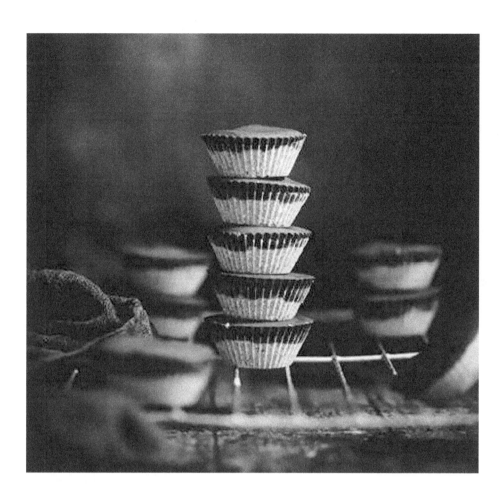

INGREDIENTS:

(makes 12 cups)

Peanut butter layer:

½ cup roasted unsalted peanuts or almonds (73 g/ 2.6 oz)

1 Tbsp coconut butter (16 g/ 0.5 oz)

¼ cup cashews or 2 Tbsp cashew 1 Tbsp Sukrin Gold, Erythritol or Swerve (10 g/ 0.4 oz)

1 heaped Tbsp almond flour (8 g/ 0.3 oz)

Blueberry jelly layer:

125 g fresh or frozen blueberries (4.4 oz)

2-5 drops liquid stevia, or to taste

Optional: gelatin powder for a firmer jelly (see tips above for details)

Chocolate layer:

8 large squares 85% dark chocolate (80 g/ 2.8 oz)

DIRECTIONS:

01. To make the base, add all ingredients into a food processor and pulse until combined and resembling a thick (but lumpy!) paste.

02. Divide evenly among 12 mini muffin molds and press down firmly (about 12 g/ 0.4 oz per cup). Place in the freezer whilst you make the jelly layer.

03. To make the jelly, add the blueberries to the food processor and mix until smooth. Add a few drops of stevia, blend, and then taste and add another drop or two if required.

04. Distribute evenly among the molds on top of the peanut base (slightly less than 1 tbsp per cup). Place in the freezer whilst you make the chocolate layer.

05. To make the chocolate top, chop the chocolate into smaller pieces and melt in a saucepan over the lowest heat.

06. Pour evenly across the jelly layer (about 1 1/2 tsp per cup) and set in the freezer at least twenty minutes.

07. Remove from the freezer and allow to sit at room temperature a few minutes before serving.

NUTRITION:

Net carbs 3.9 g

Protein 3.1 g

Fat 8.5 g

Calories 103 kcal

Total carbs 5.5 g

Fiber 1.6 g

Sugars 2.4 g

Saturated fat 3.2 g

Sodium 3 mg (0% RDA)

Magnesium 35 mg (9% RDA)

Potassium 122 mg (6% EMR)

RASPBERRY PUDDING BOWL

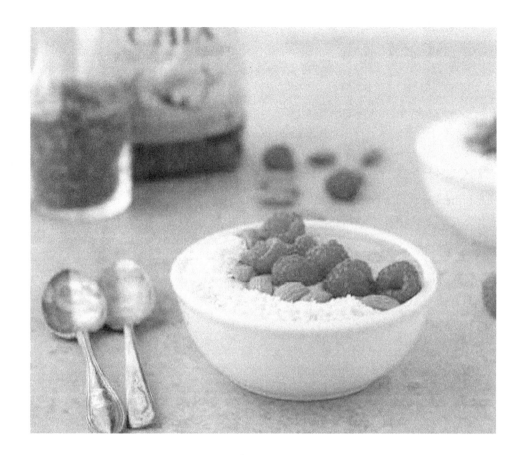

PREP TIME: 5 MINUTES

SERVES: 3

INGREDIENTS:

Breakfast Pudding

1 ½ cup full-fat coconut milk

(350 ml)

1 cup frozen raspberries

(110 grams)

¼ cup MCT oil

2 Tbsp Bob's Red Mill Chia Seeds

1 Tbsp apple cider vinegar

1 tsp alcohol-free vanilla extract

3 drops alcohol-free stevia

Optional Toppings

Shredded coconut

Almonds

Hemp hearts

Fresh berries

DIRECTIONS:

Place all of the breakfast pudding ingredients in the jug of your blender or bowl of your food processor. Blend until smooth. Divide between 3 bowls at least ¾ cup (180 ml) in size. Top with your favorite toppings, if using.

NUTRITION:

Calories 328

Calories from Fat 307.8

Total Fat 34.2 g

Saturated Fat 30.8 g

Sodium 26 mg

Carbs 8.8 g

Dietary Fiber 3.1 g

Net Carbs 5.7 g

Sugars 3.4 g

Protein 3.2 g

KETO CHICKEN ENCHILADA

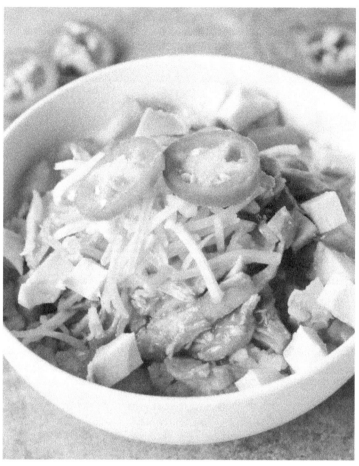

This Keto Chicken Enchilada Bowl is a low carb twist on a Mexican favorite! It's SO easy to make, totally filling and ridiculously yummy!

YIELD: 4 SERVINGS

INGREDIENTS:

2 Tbsp coconut oil (for searing chicken)

1 lb of boneless, skinless chicken thighs

¾ cup red enchilada sauce (recipe from Low Carb Maven)

¼ cup water

¼ cup chopped onion

1–4 oz can diced green chilies

Toppings (feel free to customize)

1 whole avocado, diced

1 cup shredded cheese (I used mild cheddar)

¼ cup chopped pickled jalapenos

½ cup sour cream

1 roma tomato, chopped

Optional: serve over plain cauliflower rice (or Mexican cauliflower rice) for a more complete meal!

DIRECTIONS:

01. In a pot or ditch oven over medium heat melt the coconut oil. Once hot, sear chicken thighs until lightly brown.

02. Pour in enchilada sauce and water then add onion and green chilies. Reduce heat to a simmer and cover. Cook chicken for 17-25 minutes or until chicken is tender and fully cooked through to at least 165 degrees internal temperature.

03. Carefully remove the chicken and place onto a work surface. Chop or shred chicken (your preference) then add it back into the pot. Let the chicken simmer uncovered for an additional 10 minutes to absorb flavor and allow the sauce to reduce a little.

04. To serve, top with avocado, cheese, jalapeno, sour cream, tomato, and any other desired toppings. Feel free to customize these to your preference. Serve alone or over cauliflower rice if desired just be sure to update your personal nutrition info as needed.

NUTRITION:

Calories 568

Fat 40.21 g

Net Carbs 6.14g

Protein 38.38 g

SKILLET CHICKEN RECIPE

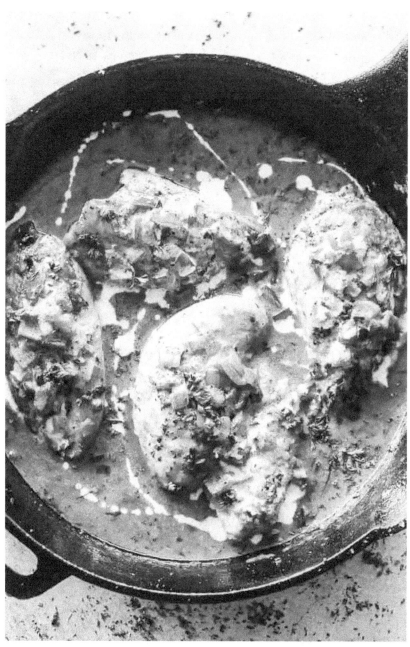

Quick and easy skillet seared chicken topped with a creamy garlic and onions white wine sauce that's sure to please any crowd!

SERVINGS: 4 SERVINGS

INGREDIENTS:

For The Chicken

1 Tbsp olive oil

4 boneless skinless chicken breasts

Salt and fresh ground pepper to taste

1 tsp garlic powder

For The Creamy White Wine Sauce

1 Tbsp unsalted butter

1 large yellow onion diced

3 garlic cloves minced salt and fresh ground pepper to taste

1 cup dry white wine

1 tsp dried thyme

½ cup half and half/heavy cream/or evaporated milk Fresh

Chopped parsley

DIRECTIONS:

For The Chicken

01. Heat olive oil in a large skillet over medium heat until the oil shimmers, about 2 to 3 minutes.

02. Season chicken with salt, pepper and garlic powder.

03. Add chicken to the skillet and cook until golden brown, about 6 minutes. DO NOT move it around.

04. Using tongs flip the chicken over and continue to cook for 6 more minutes, or until cooked through.

05. Remove chicken from skillet to a plate; cover and set aside.

For The Creamy White Wine Sauce

01. DO NOT wipe the skillet.

02. Add butter to skillet and melt over medium-high heat.

03. Add onions and cook for 3 minutes, or until softened.

04. Stir in garlic, salt, and pepper; cook for 30 seconds, or until fragrant.

05. Add wine and bring to a simmer, scraping the bottom of the skillet to mix the brown bits into the liquid; cook for 4 to 5 more minutes, or until half of the wine has reduced.

06. Stir in thyme and half-and-half.

07. Reduce heat to slowly bring to a boil; place chicken breasts back in the skillet and leave to simmer and thicken for about 4 minutes.

08. Remove skillet from heat.

09. Garnish with fresh chopped parsley.

10. Serve.

NUTRITION:

Calories 276

Calories from Fat 90

Total Fat 10 g

Saturated Fat 3 g

Cholesterol 85 mg

Sodium 151 mg

Potassium 520 mg

Total Carbohydrates 6 g

Dietary Fiber 0 g

Sugars 2 g

Protein 25 g

EASY KETO BREAKFAST

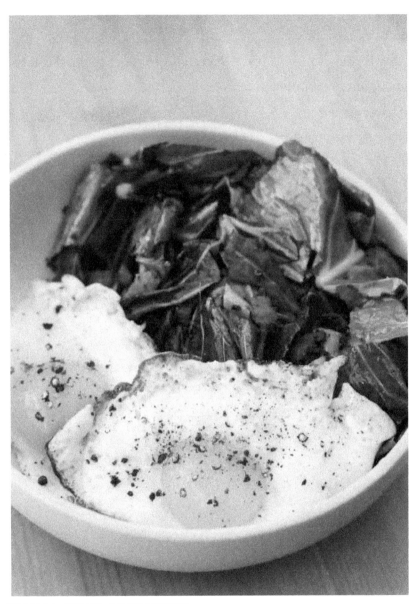

TOTAL TIME: 5 MINUTES

SERVINGS: 1 BOWL

INGREDIENTS:

2 large eggs

3 slices bacon

3 cups collard greens

¼ tsp black pepper

½ tsp Pink Himalayan Salt

¼ tsp garlic powder

½ Tbsp ghee

DIRECTIONS:

01. Heat a large skillet to medium-high heat and slice up the bacon into pieces. Add the bacon to the hot pan and allow to cook down.

02. Once the bacon is cooked to your liking add in the collard greens and season with garlic powder, salt and pepper. Cook the collards down to your liking and then transfer bacon and collards to a bowl.

03. Add the ghee to the hot pan and crack in the eggs. Let them fry up until the white is fully cooked through and season them with salt and pepper. Once the eggs are cooked add them to your bowl and enjoy!

NUTRITION:

Calories 402kcal

Carbohydrates 7g

Protein 24g

Fat 33g

Fiber 4g

PAN FRIED FISH WITH BUTTER SAUCE

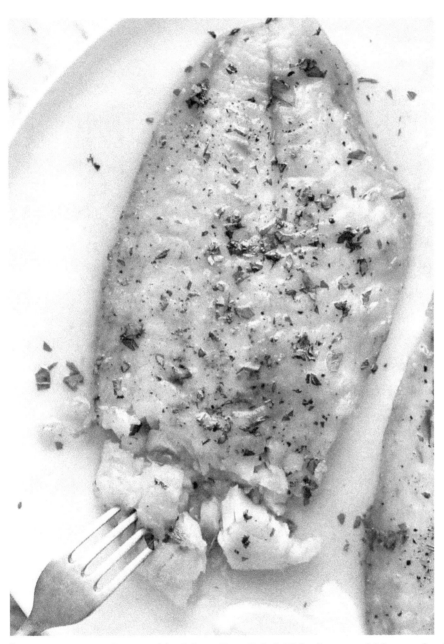

A Lemon Butter Sauce with Crispy Pan Fried Fish that would be perfectly at home in a posh restaurant yet is so quick to make at home! Browning the butter gives the sauce a rich, nutty aroma which pairs beautifully with fresh lemon, as well as thickening the sauce and giving it a gorgeous golden color.

INGREDIENTS:

Lemon Butter Sauce:

60 g / 4 Tbsp unsalted butter , cut into pieces

1 Tbsp fresh lemon juice

Salt and finely ground pepper

Crispy Pan Fried Fish:

2 x thin white fish fillets (120-150g / 4-5oz each), skinless boneless

Salt and pepper

2 Tbsp white flour

2 Tbsp oil (I use canola)

Serving:

Lemon wedges Finely chopped parsley, optional

DIRECTIONS:

Lemon Butter Sauce

01. Place the butter in a light colored saucepan or small skillet over medium heat.

02. Melt butter then leave on the stove, whisking / stirring very now and then. When the butter turns golden brown and it smells nutty — about 3 minutes, remove from stove immediately and pour into small bowl. (Note 2)

03. Add lemon juice and a pinch of salt and pepper. Stir then taste when it has cooled slightly. Adjust lemon/salt to taste.

04. Set aside — it will stay pourable for 20 — 30 minutes.

Crispy Pan Fried Fish:

01. Pat fish dry using paper towels. Sprinkle with salt & pepper, then flour. Use fingers to spread flour. Turn and repeat. Shake excess flour off well, slapping between hands if necessary.

02. Heat oil in a non stick skillet over high heat. When the oil is shimmering and there are faint wisps of smoke, add fish. Cook for 1 1/2 minutes until golden and crispy on the edges, then turn and cook the other side for 1 1/2 minutes (cook longer if you

have thicker fillets).

03. Remove immediately onto serving plates. Drizzle each with about 1 tbsp of Sauce (avoid dark specks settled at the bottom of the bowl), garnish with parsley and serve with lemon on the side. Pictured in post with Kale and Quinoa Salad.

NUTRITION:

Calories 393

Total fat 28 g

Cholesterol 127 mg

Sodium 464 mg

Potassium 518 mg

Total Carbohydrate 3.1 g

Protein 31 g

CHICKEN SATAY RECIPE WITH PEANUT SAUCE

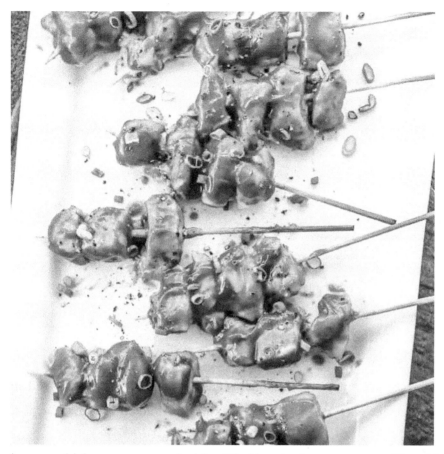

An easy chicken satay served with a Thai inspired peanut sauce. The chicken is soaked in a coconut milk marinade before baking in the oven or grilling.

SERVINGS 4 SERVINGS

INGREDIENTS:

2 boneless skinless chicken breasts (¾ to 1 pound total)

10 wooden skewers soaked for about 30 minutes before using

1 scallion thinly sliced

Marinade:

½ cup full-fat coconut milk

3 cloves garlic minced

½ tsp curry powder

½ tsp salt

½ tsp ground black pepper

¼ tsp cayenne powder

Peanut sauce:

¼ cup natural creamy peanut butter

3 cloves garlic minced

2 Tbsp sesame oil

1 Tbsp olive oil

1 Tbsp soy sauce

1 Tbsp lime juice

NUTRITION:

Calories 330

Total Fat 20 g

Saturated Fat 3 g

Trans Fat 0 g

Cholesterol 66 mg

Sodium 500 mg

Potassium 300 mg

Total Carb 5 g

Dietary Fiber 2 g

Sugars 1.5 g

Protein 30 g

DIRECTIONS:

01. Marinating the chicken: In a large bowl, combine all marinade ingredients and stir until well-mixed. Cut chicken breasts into 1 inch chunks and add them to the marinade, stirring to coat well. Cover and refrigerate for at least 6 hours.

02. Cooking the chicken: Thread chicken chunks onto the skewers, leaving about half of each skewer empty for handling. Place them in a single layer on a large baking sheet. Bake at 450 F for 10 minutes, flip the skewers, and then bake another 5 minutes or until cooked through. Alternatively, you can grill the chicken skewers.

03. Making the sauce: While waiting for the chicken to cook, add all peanut sauce ingredients to a small saucepan. Whisk together over medium-low heat until smooth, a few minutes. Keep warm over low heat, stirring occasionally.

04. Serving: Transfer chicken skewers onto a serving plate. Brush peanut sauce over the chicken. Top with sliced scallions and optionally black pepper. Serve while warm.

LOW CARB CHICKEN POT PIE

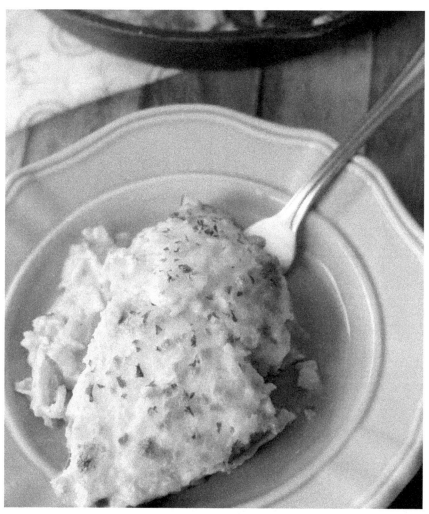

If you want comfort foods, look no further than this Keto Low Carb Chicken Pot Pie Recipe! This will totally wow your family, and will satisfy your cravings. So much flavor and so easy to make!

SERVINGS: 8 SERVINGS

INGREDIENTS:

For the Chicken Pot Pie Filling:

2 Tbsp of butter

½ cup mixed veggies could also substitute green beans or broccoli

¼ small onion diced

¼ tsp pink salt

¼ tsp pepper

2 garlic cloves minced

¾ cup heavy whipping cream

1 cup chicken broth

1 tsp poultry seasoning

¼ tsp rosemary pinch thyme

2 ½ cups cooked chicken diced

¼ tsp Xanthan Gum

For the crust:

4 ½ Tbsp of butter melted and cooled

⅓ cup coconut flour

2 Tbsp full fat sour cream

4 eggs

¼ tsp salt

¼ tsp baking powder

1 ⅓ cup sharp shredded cheddar cheese or mozzarella shredded

DIRECTIONS:

01. Cook 1 to 1 1/2 lbs chicken in the slow cooker for 3 hours on high or 6 hours on low.

02. Preheat oven to 400 degrees.

03. Sautee onion, mixed veggies, garlic cloves, salt, and pepper in 2 tablespoons butter in an oven safe skillet for approx 5 min or until onions are translucent.

04. Add heavy whipping cream, chicken broth, poultry seasoning, thyme, and rosemary.

05. Sprinkle Xanthan Gum on top and simmer for 5 minutes so that the sauce thickens. Make sure to simmer covered as the liquid will evaporate otherwise. You need a lot of liquid for this

recipe, otherwise, it will be dry.

06. Add diced chicken.

07. Make the breading by combining melted butter (I cool mine by popping the bowl in the fridge for 5 min), eggs, salt, and sour cream in a bowl then whisk together.

08. Add coconut flour and baking powder to the mixture and stir until combined.

09. Stir in cheese.

10. Drop batter by dollops on top of the chicken pot pie. Do not spread it out, as the coconut flour will absorb too much of the liquid.

11. Bake in a 400-degree oven for 15-20 min.

12. Set oven to broil and move chicken pot pie to top shelf. Broil for 1-2 minutes until bread topping is nicely browned. Sprinkle a little dried parsley on top if desired.

NUTRITION:

Calories 297 kcal

Carbohydrates 5.3 g

Protein 11.6 g

Fat 17 g

Fiber 2 g

STUFFED AVOCADOS WITH CHICKEN SALAD

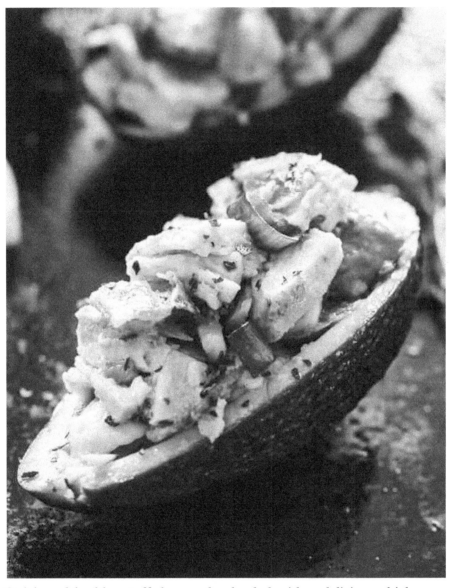

Quick and healthy stuffed avocados loaded with a delicious chicken, avocado, and bacon salad tossed in a refreshing lemon dressing. Perfect keto lunch idea!

SERVINGS: 6 SERVINGS

INGREDIENTS:

For The Stuffed Avocados:

12 slices low sodium turkey bacon or low sodium bacon

3 whole avocados, cut in half, pits removed

½ lemon

2 cups diced or shredded baked chicken breasts OR rotisserie chicken

3 green onions, washed, trimmed, and sliced (keep the sliced green parts for garnish)

plain nonfat yogurt or low fat sour cream, optional

dried parsley, for garnish, optional

cracked black pepper, for garnish, optional

For The Lemon Dressing:

¼ cup extra virgin olive oil

¼ cup fresh lemon juice

½ tsp dried oregano

1 clove garlic, minced

Salt and fresh ground pepper, to taste

DIRECTIONS:

For The Stuffed Avocados

01. Cook the bacon to a desired crispness; when cool enough to handle, crumble it into a salad bowl.

02. Cut the avocados, remove the pits, and carefully scoop out the flesh.

03. Dice up the avocado flesh and add it to the salad bowl.

04. Squeeze a bit of lemon juice over the diced avocados and the empty avocado shells to prevent from browning.

05. in the salad bowl, mix in the diced or shredded chicken and the white part of the sliced green onions. Set aside.

For The Lemon Dressing

01. Whisk together all of the ingredients in a small bowl; adjust the seasonings to taste and pour it over the salad.

02. Taste the salad and adjust the seasonings.

03. Using a spoon, scoop out the prepared chicken bacon salad and fill the empty avocado shells.

04. If desired, add a dollop of plain nonfat yogurt or sour cream.

05. Garnish with sliced green onions, dried parsley and cracked black pepper.

06. Serve.

NUTRITION:

Calories 215

Calories from Fat 126

Total Fat 14 g

Saturated Fat 3 g

Cholesterol 59 mg

Sodium 196 mg

Potassium 210 mg

Total Carbohydrates 2 g

Protein 18 g

SPINACH ARTICHOKE STUFFED CHICKEN BREAST

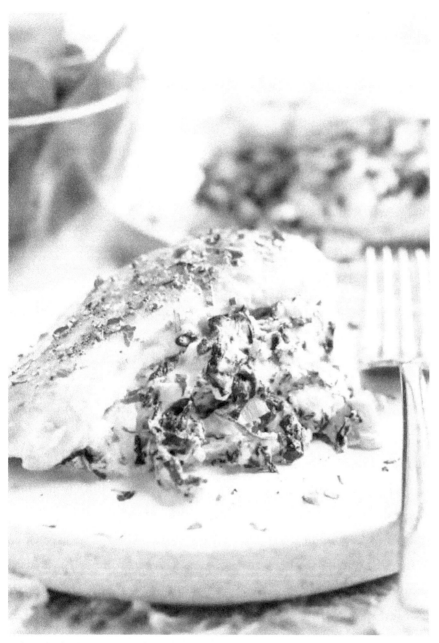

Spinach Artichoke Stuffed Chicken Breast is the perfect combination of your favorite dip and favorite bird, all rolled into one quick and easy Ketogenic stuffed chicken breast recipe! These spinach and mozzarella stuffed chicken breasts are gluten-free, lowcarb, and Keto diet-approved!

SERVINGS 6 SERVINGS

INGREDIENTS:

1 ½ lbs chicken breasts 6 4-oz. portions

2 Tbsp olive oil

4 oz cream cheese softened

¼ cup Greek yogurt

½ cup Mozzarella cheese shredded

½ cup artichoke hearts thinly sliced

¼ cup frozen spinach drained, and tightly packed

½ tsp salt divided

¼ tsp pepper divided

NUTRITION:

Calories 288

Calories from Fat 153

Total Fat 17 g

Saturated Fat 6 g

Cholesterol 101 mg

Sodium 481 mg

Potassium 486 mg

Total Carbohydrates 2 g

Sugars 1 g

Protein 28 g

DIRECTIONS:

01. Pound chicken breast to 1-inch thick. Using a sharp knife cut each chicken breast down the middle, being careful not to cut all of the way through, to make a pocket for the spinach artichoke filling. Sprinkle chicken breasts with ¼ teaspoon salt and 1/8 teaspoon pepper.

02. In a medium-sized bowl combine the cream cheese, Greek yogurt, Mozzarella cheese, artichoke hearts, drained spinach, ¼ teaspoon salt and 1/8 teaspoon pepper. Mix until thoroughly combined.

03. Carefully fill each chicken breast with equal amounts of the spinach artichoke filling. If you have extra filling, set it aside until the chicken is almost done cooking.

04. In a large skillet over medium heat add olive oil and stuffed chicken breasts. Cover skillet and cook for 7-8 minutes on each side, or until chicken reaches 165 degrees with a meat thermometer.

05. During the last few minutes of cooking, add additional filling to the skillet to heat it up. Serve chicken with cauliflower rice, regular rice, mashed cauliflower, or mashed potatoes and enjoy!

KETO BROCCOLI SALAD

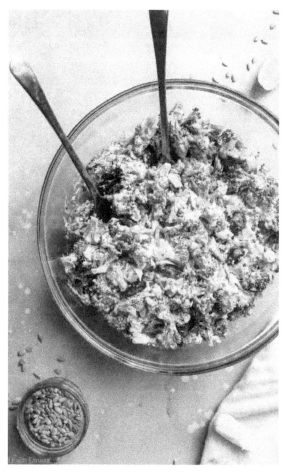

This Mediterranean Low Carb Broccoli Salad is a super easy, healthy and protein packed side dish for dinner or a potluck! It's made with Greek yogurt and you won't even miss the mayo!

SERVINGS 8 PEOPLE, AS A SIDE

INGREDIENTS:

For the salad:

5 cups Broccoli, cut into small florets (380g)

½ cup Artichoke hearts marinated in olive oil, sliced

½ cup Sun-dried tomatoes in olive oil, roughly chopped (75g) (oil squeezed out)

½ cup Pitted Kalamata olives, halved

⅓ cup Red onion, diced

¼ cup Roasted salted sunflower seeds

For the dressing:

2 cups Plain, non-fat Greek yogurt Zest and juice of 1 large lemon

4 ½ tsp Monk fruit (or granulated sweetener of choice)

1 ¾ tsp Dried oregano

1 ½ tsp Fresh garlic, minced

1 ½ tsp Dried ground basil

1 ½ tsp Dried ground thyme

1 tsp Sea salt Pepper

2 Tbsp Oil from the jar of sun-dried tomatoes

DIRECTIONS:

01. In a large bowl, mix together ALL of the salad ingredients.

02. In a medium bowl, stir together all of the dressing ingredients.

03. Pour the dressing over the broccoli and stir to coat well. Cover and refrigerate for at least 2 hours, up to overnight, so that broccoli can absorb the dressing and develop the flavor. 0

4. DEVOUR!

NUTRITION:

Calories 182

Calories from Fat 112

Total Fat 12.4 g

Saturated Fat 0.9 g

Polyunsaturated Fat 1.7 g

Monounsaturated Fat 2.9 g

Cholesterol 2.5 mg

Sodium 365 mg

Potassium 212 mg

Total Carbohydrates 14.7 g

Dietary Fiber 3.6 g

Sugars 5.9 g

Protein 5.9 g

CHEESY OMELETTE

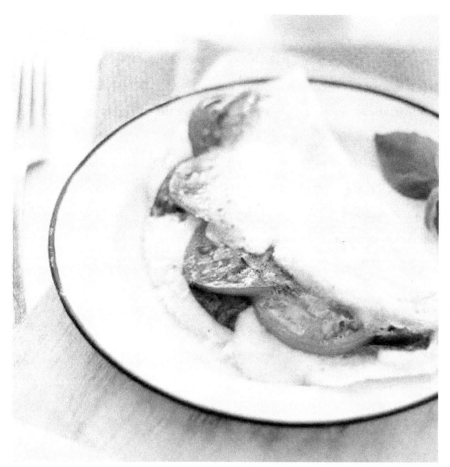

A delicious and easy low carb omelette recipe that will have you looking forward to mornings! Keto and Atkins friendly!

INGREDIENTS:

2 eggs

1 Tbsp water

1 Tbsp butter

3 thin slices deli Sopressata (you can sub in salami or prosciutto if that's what you have)

6 fresh basil leaves

5 thin slices fresh, ripe tomato

2 oz fresh mozzarella cheese

Salt and pepper to taste

DIRECTIONS:

01. Whisk together the eggs and water in a small bowl.

02. Melt the butter in a nonstick sauté pan over low to medium heat.

03. Pour in the egg mixture and cook for 30 seconds.

04. Spread the meat slices on one half of the egg mixture. Top with the cheese, tomatoes, and basil slices. Season with salt and pepper.

05. Cook for about 2 minutes or until the empty half of the egg mixture is firm enough to fold over the ingredients. Use a spatula to gently fold the omelette in half.

06. Cover the pan and cook on low heat for another minute or two or until the omelette is cooked through and there is no raw egg left in the middle.

07. To remove, tilt the pan and slide the omelette gently out onto a plate.

NUTRITION:

Calories 451

Fat 36 g

Net Carbs 3 g

Protein 33 g

LOW-CARB RAINBOW CHARD & SAUSAGE HASH

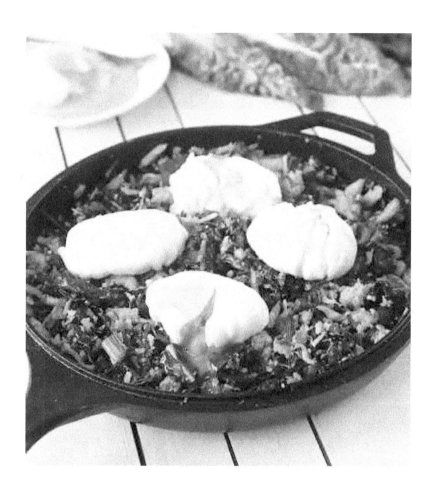

INGREDIENTS:

200 g Swiss chard or dark-leaf kale (7.1 oz)

2 cups cauli-rice (240 g/ 8.5 oz)

150 g gluten-free sausage meat (5.3 oz)

3 Tbsp ghee or lard, you can make your own ghee (45 g/ 1.6 oz)

2 cloves garlic

1 Tbsp fresh lemon juice

1 tsp Dijon mustard (you can make your own)

Sea salt and black pepper, to taste

Top with 4 poached eggs

DIRECTIONS:

01. Start by preparing the vegetables. You can find details on how to "rice" the cauliflower here. When done, set aside.

02. Then cut the stalks of the chard off and chop into small pieces.

03. Place the sausage meat in a large pan greased with a tablespoon of the ghee and cook until browned from all sides. When cooked, use a slotted spoon to transfer into a bowl.

04. Add the remaining ghee to the pan. Peel and finely chop the garlic and place into the pan. Cook for just about a minute or until fragrant. Then, add the cauli-rice and cook over a medium heat for 5 minutes. Stir to prevent burning.

05. Then add the chard stalks, Dijon mustard,

06. Lemon juice, and cook for another 2 minutes while stirring. Season with salt and pepper to taste and mix until well combined.

07. Meanwhile, roughly chop the chard leaves and add to the pan. Cook for another 2 minutes. 08. When done, add the cooked sausage, mix and take off the heat. Top with poached or fried eggs.

NUTRITION:

Net carbs 8.3 g

Protein 29.4 g

Fat 46 g

Calories 576 kcal

Total carbs 12.8 grams

Fiber 4.6 grams

Sugars 4.3 grams

Saturated fat 21.7 grams

Sodium 789 mg (34% RDA)

Magnesium 125 mg (31% RDA)

Potassium 1,098 mg (55% EMR)

PESTO SCRAMBLED EGGS

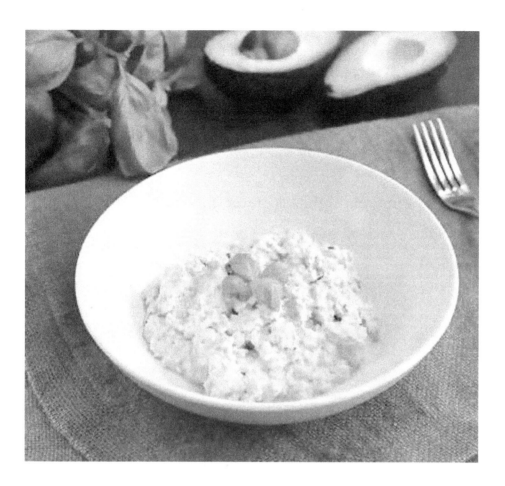

INGREDIENTS:

3 large eggs, free-range or organic

1 Tbsp butter or ghee, grass-fed. You can make your own ghee – basil or garlic infused ghee work great! (15g / 0.5 oz)

1 Tbsp pesto (you can make your own green pesto or red pesto) (15g / 0.5 oz)

2 Tbsp crème fraîche or soured cream or creamed coconut milk (30g / 1.1 oz)

Salt to taste

Freshly ground black pepper to taste

DIRECTIONS:

01. Crack the eggs into a mixing bowl with a pinch of salt and pepper and beat them well with a whisk or fork.

02. Pour the eggs into a pan, add butter or ghee and turn the heat on.

03. Keep on low heat while stirring constantly. Do not stop stirring as the eggs may get dry and lose the creamy texture. Add the pesto and mix in well.

04. Take off the heat, spoon crème fraîche in and mix well with the eggs.

05. This will help the eggs cool down and stop cooking while keeping the creamy texture.

06. Place on a serving plate and try with sliced avocado on top.

NUTRITION:

Net carbs 2.6 g

Protein 20.4 g

Fat 41.5 g

Calories 468 kcal

Total carbs 3.3 g

Fiber 0.7 g

Sugars 1.4 g

Saturated fat 19.5 g

Sodium 874 mg (38% RDA)

Magnesium 26 mg (6% RDA)

Potassium 327 mg (16% EMR)

HOMEMADE MAPLE SAGE BREAKFAST SAUSAGES

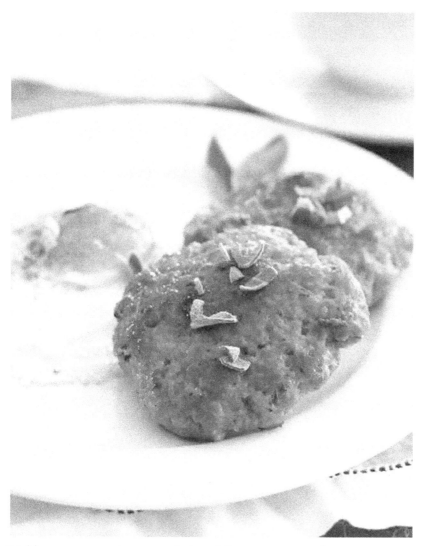

Making your own homemade breakfast sausage patties means you can skip the added sugars but still get all the great flavor!

INGREDIENTS:

1 lb ground pork

2 Tbsp chopped fresh sage

2 Tbsp granular Swerve Sweetener

1 tsp maple extract

1 tsp salt

½ tsp pepper

¼ tsp garlic powder

⅛ tsp cayenne

DIRECTIONS:

01. In a large bowl, combine pork, sage, Swerve, maple, salt, pepper, garlic powder and cayenne. Use hands to mix thoroughly. Form into 8 even patties and flatten to about 1 inch thick.

02. Add a little oil or butter to a large skillet over medium heat. Add patties and cook about 3 to 4 minutes per side, until an instant read thermometer inserted in the center reaches 145F.

03. Makes about 4 servings.

NUTRITION:

Food energy 257 kcal

Saturated fatty acids 7.31 g

Total fat 17.79 g

Calories from fat 160

Cholesterol 65 mg

Carbohydrate 0.34 g

Total dietary fiber 0.51 g

Protein 17.65 g

Sodium 647 mg

KETO MUG MUFFIN

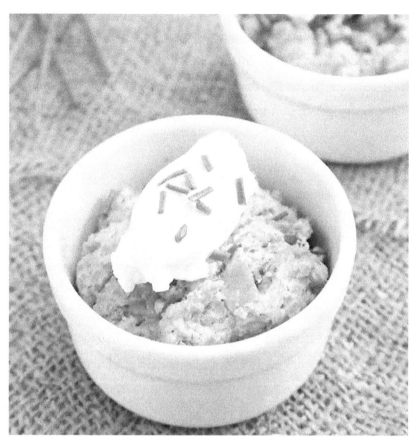

Mug muffins and mug cakes are some of the most convenient keto-friendly meals. They can be made both sweet and savory and take just a few minutes to prepare. For those of you that may not have a microwave, I included some tips for baking the muffins in the oven.

INGREDIENTS: (makes 2 servings)

Basic savory mug muffin mix:
 ¼ cup almond flour (25 g / 0.9 oz)
 ¼ cup flax meal (38 g / 1.3 oz)
 ¼ tsp baking soda
 1 large egg, free-range or organic
 2 Tbsp cream or coconut milk

2 Tbsp water pinch salt

Add: 60 g smoked salmon (2.1 oz) 2 Tbsp freshly chopped chives or spring onion serve with 2 dollops full-fat cream cheese or sour cream (60 g / 2.1 oz) If you need to make this recipe nut free, use more flax meal (same amount) or coconut flour (half the amount). When using ingredients, always go by their weight, especially in case of baked goods. Measures such as cups may vary depending on a product / brand. When looking for ingredients, try to get them in their most natural form (organic, without unnecessary additives).

DIRECTIONS:

01. Place all the dry ingredients in a small bowl and combine well.

02. Add the egg, cream, water and mix well using a fork.

03. Slice the smoked salmon and finely chop the chives. Add to the mixture and combine well. 04. Microwave on high for 60-90 seconds. When done, top with a dollop of cream cheese and enjoy!

05. Tips for cooking in the oven: If you don't have a microwave, I suggest you make 4-8 servings at once. Preheat the oven to 175 °C/ 350 °F and cook for about 12-15 minutes or until cooked in the centre.

NUTRITION:

Net carbs 3 g

Protein 17.2 g

Fat 32.3 g

Calories 374 kcal

Total carbs 9.5 g

Fiber 6.5 g

Sugars 2.4 g

Saturated fat 11.3 g

Sodium 553 mg (24% RDA)

Magnesium 120 mg (30% RDA)

Potassium 383 mg (19% EMR)

STUFFED MANICOTTI

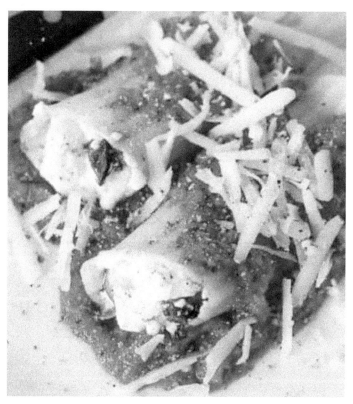

SERVING: 6

INGREDIENTS:

1 large eggplant

1 package organic Chicken Sausage

1 ½ cups cottage cheese

2 cups shredded mozzarella cheese

½ cup grated Parmesan cheese

2 egg whites

½ tsp dried oregano

1 (32 oz) jar no sugar marinara sauce

DIRECTIONS:

01. To prepare the shells, peel eggplant and cut into long "lasagna noodle" like shapes. Make a cylinder and pin with toothpicks. Chop the chicken sausage into very small pieces.

02. Preheat oven to 350 degrees F (175 degrees C). Combine sausage, cottage cheese, 1 cup mozzarella cheese, Parmesan cheese, egg whites and oregano. Mix well. Stuff "shells" with mixture.

03. Lightly grease a 9×13 inch baking dish. Pour enough spaghetti sauce in dish to cover the bottom. Place stuffed "shells" in the dish. Cover with pasta sauce and top with the remaining 1 cup mozzarella cheese. Bake in preheated oven for 50 minutes.

NUTRITION:

Traditional Manicotti

Calories 611

Fat 15 g

Protein 40 g

Carbs 43.2

Fiber 3.7 g

"Healthified" Manicotti

Calories 385

Fat 15 g

Protein 40 g

Carbs 5.2

Fiber 3.5 g

BACON AND CARAMELIZED ONION SMOTHERED PORK CHOPS

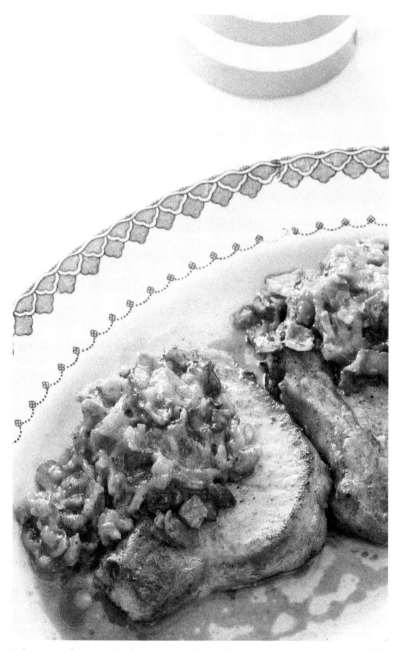

Juicy, tender pork chops smothered in a creamy onion and bacon sauce. This might be the best low carb meal I've ever had!

SERVINGS: 4 CHOPS

INGREDIENTS:

6 slices bacon chopped

2 small onions thinly sliced

¼ tsp salt

¼ pepper

4 bone-in pork chops

1 inch thick

Salt and pepper to taste

½ cup chicken broth

¼ cup heavy cream

NUTRITION:

Carbs 6.3 g

Fiber 1.02 g

Total Net Carbs 5.28 g

Food energy 352 kcal

Saturated fatty acids 8.43 g

Total fat 18.23 g

Calories from fat 164

Cholesterol 107 mg

Carbohydrate 6.30 g

Total dietary fiber 1.02 g

Protein 36.98 g

Sodium 725 mg

DIRECTIONS:

01. In a large sauté pan, cook bacon over medium heat until crisp. Use a slotted spoon to remove to a bowl, reserving bacon grease.

02. Add onions to bacon grease and sprinkle with salt and pepper. Cook, stirring frequently, for 15 to 20 minutes, until onions are soft and golden brown. Add onions to bacon in the bowl.

03. Increase heat to medium high and sprinkle pork chops with salt and pepper. Add chops to pan and brown on the first

side 3 minutes. Then turn chops over and reduce heat to medium, cooking on the second side until internal temperature reaches 135F, about 7 to 10 more minutes. Remove to a platter and tent with foil.

04. Add broth to pan and scrape up any browned bits. Add cream and simmer until mixture is thickened, 2 or 3 minutes. Return onions and bacon to pan and stir to combine. 05. Top pork chops with onion and bacon mixture and serve.

CHICKEN TACOS

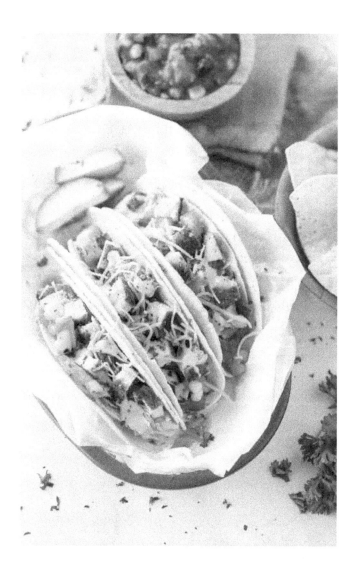

INGREDIENTS: (makes 2 servings)

1 package chicken thighs, skinned, boneless (400g / 14.1 oz / 0.88 lbs)

½ medium red onion (50g / 1.8 oz)

½ lime, juiced

2 cloves garlic

1 Tbsp fresh thyme (or ½ tsp dried thyme)

1 Tbsp fresh oregano (or ½ tsp dried oregano)

½ tsp paprika

¼ tsp cayenne pepper

2 Tbsp ghee or butter fresh full-fat cream or coconut milk (60 ml / 2 fl oz)

salt and pepper to taste

2 heads small lettuce (200g / 7.1 oz)

DIRECTIONS:

01. Peel, halve and finely chop the onion, mash the garlic and chop the herbs (if you are using fresh herbs).

02. Dice the chicken thighs, mix with garlic, herbs, paprika, cayenne and black pepper and season with salt. Squeeze in the lime juice. Note: I prefer using chicken thighs to breast filets. They are a lot juicier and tender!

03. Heat a large skillet, add ghee or butter and cook the onion over medium heat until it becomes soft and golden.

04. add the herbed chicken pieces and cook for about 10 minutes or until done.

05. Keep on medium heat, add the cream and let it cook for another 2-3 minutes while stirring frequently. When done, set aside.

06. Wash the lettuce (I used Little Gem lettuce) and place in a salad spinner or drain using a paper towel. Spoon the meat mixture on top of each leaf and enjoy! :-)

NUTRITION:

Net carbs 6.4 g

Protein 41.4 g

Fat 35.4 g

Calories 525 kcal

Total carbs 9 g

Fiber 2.6 g

Sugars 3.2 g

Saturated fat 18.5 g

Sodium 808 mg (35% RDA)

Magnesium 70 mg (17% RDA)

Potassium 810 mg (41% EMR)

CHORIZO MEATBALLS

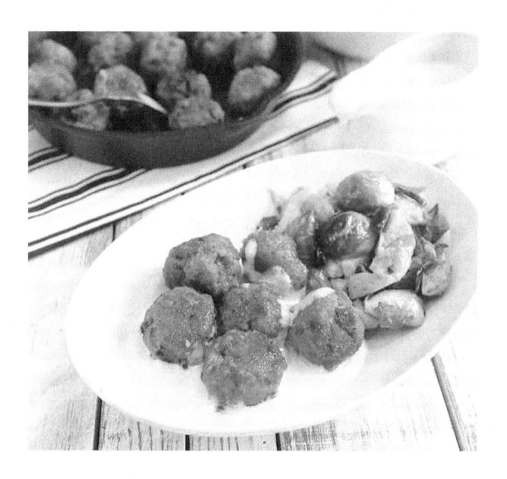

INGREDIENTS:

(makes 4 servings)

0.9 lb ground pork, 20% fat (400 g / 14.1 oz)

⅓ Average Spanish chorizo or other hard type (80 g / 2.8 oz)

1 large egg, free-range or organic

½ cup almond flour (50 g / 1.8 oz)

1 tsp paprika

¼ tsp cayenne pepper

1 tsp ground cumin

2 cloves garlic

1 small white onion (70 g / 2.5 oz)

1 Tbsp ghee or lard (make your own ghee)

½ tsp salt

DIRECTIONS:

01. Peel and dice the onion and garlic and dice the chorizo sausage.

02. Grease a large pan with ghee and add the chorizo, garlic and onion. Cook for 5-8 minutes over a medium heat or until lightly crisped up. Take off the heat and set aside.

03. In a mixing bowl, combine the ground pork, egg, almond flour, paprika, cayenne pepper, ground cumin and salt.

04. Mix until well combined and add the crisped up chorizo, garlic and onion from the pan using a slotted spoon.

05. Using your hands, make small-medium meatballs and place on a cutting board.

06. Heat the pan where you cooked the chorizo and onion over a medium-high heat. Once hot, add the meatballs and cook for 2 minutes.

07. Once browned, turn the meatballs on the other side using a fork and cook for another 2 minutes. Reduce the heat to medium and cook for 5-10 minutes. The time depends on the size of the meatballs.

08. Remove from the heat and serve immediately or let it cool down and store in the fridge for up to 5 days. To store them for longer, place in a zip-lock bag and freeze.

NUTRITION:

Net carbs 4.1 g

Protein 27.5 g

Fat 35.4 g

Calories 448 kcal

Total carbs 6 g

Fiber 1.9 g

Sugars 1.5 g

Saturated fat 11 g

Sodium 625 mg (27% RDA)

Magnesium 61 mg (15% RDA)

Potassium 507 mg (25% EMR)

LOW CARB KETO CUPCAKES

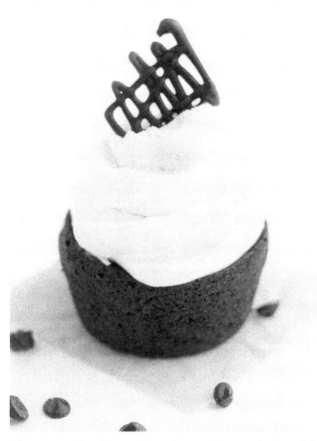

These amazing Keto Cupcakes really are the best! A moist and easy low carb chocolate cupcake recipe pulled together with just a few simple ingredients.

SERVING: 12 CUPCAKES

INGREDIENTS:

⅓ cup coconut flour

½ cup unsweetened cocoa powder

¼ cup powdered erythritol (another low carb sweetener of your choice will work)

1 tsp baking powder

½ tsp baking soda

¼ tsp salt

4 whole eggs

1 tsp vanilla extract

8 drops stevia extract optional for extra sweetness

4 Tbsp extra light olive oil

½ cup unsweetened almond milk (or another dairy-free alternative)

DIRECTIONS:

01. Preheat oven to 350 degrees F. Prepare a muffin tin by greasing or baking with cupcake liners.

02. in a medium bowl whisk together coconut flour, cocoa powder, erythritol, baking powder, baking soda, and salt.

03. Make a well in the center of dry mixture. Add eggs, vanilla extract, stevia (if adding), olive oil and almond milk. Mix until ingredients are well combined. Allow to sit for 5-8 minutes.

04. If mixture becomes thicker in consistency than you'd like feel free to add 2 Tablespoons of water to batter until it reaches your desired consistency.

05. Spoon 2 Tablespoons of batter into each tin. Bake 20-22 minutes, or until toothpick comes out clean.

06. Frost with your favorite low carb frosting and enjoy!

NUTRITION:

Calories 66

Calories from Fat 45

Total Fat 5 g

Saturated Fat 1 g

Cholesterol 1 mg

Sodium 116 mg

Potassium 88 mg

Total Carbohydrates 7 g

Dietary Fiber 2 g

Sugars 0 g

Protein 1 g

KETO CINNAMON ROLLS

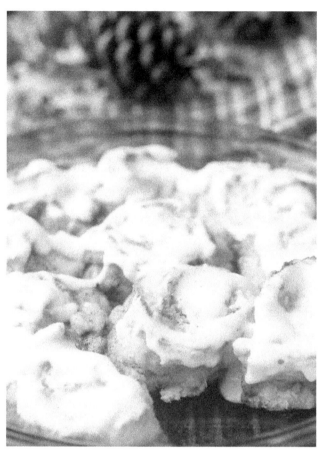

SERVING: 12

INGREDIENTS:

Dough

2 cups mozzarella cheese part skim, shredded

3 oz cream cheese

2 eggs

1 tsp vanilla extract

½ tsp vanilla liquid stevia

½ cup coconut flour

½ tsp xanthan gum

¼ tsp salt

1 Tbsp baking powder

¼ cup Swerve sweetener

Cinnamon "Sugar"

½ cup butter melted

⅓ cup Sukrin Gold or use Swerve brown sugar

2 tsp cinnamon

Cream Cheese Frosting

3 Tbsp heavy cream

3 oz cream cheese

1 Tbsp Swerve sweetener

½ tsp vanilla extract

NUTRITION:

Calories 219

Calories from Fat 171

Total Fat 19 g

Saturated Fat 11 g

Cholesterol 77 mg

Sodium 303 mg

Potassium 144 mg

Total Carbohydrates 4 g

Dietary Fiber 2 g

Sugars 1 g

Protein 6 g

DIRECTIONS:

01. Preheat the oven to 400 degrees F.

02. Combine the mozzarella and cream cheese and melt together either 2 minutes in a microwave or over the stove on low heat. Stir until smooth.

03. Add the remaining dough ingredients, wet hand and thoroughly incorporate as much as possible.

04. Roll the dough on a piece of parchment paper, top with another sheet of parchment since the dough is quite sticky, about 16 by 8 in.

05. Slice into 12 strips. Set aside.

06. Combine the melted butter, sugar free sweetener and cinnamon. Mix well to combine, use half the mixture to spread onto the strips of dough. Roll them up and place them on a greased or parchment lined pie dish. Use the remaining butter mixture to pour over the tops of the cinnamon rolls.

07. Bake 15-18 minutes. While they are baking you can make the frosting.

08. Add the frosting ingredients into a blender and blend until smooth.

09. Once rolls are hot out of the oven spread the frosting over the tops of the rolls and enjoy!

VANILLA BEAN FRAPPUCCINO

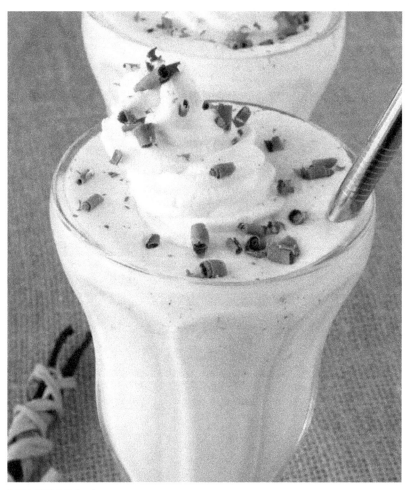

SERVINGS: 4

INGREDIENTS:

2 cups vanilla almond milk unsweetened

1 cup heavy whipping cream

1 vanilla bean or 1 tsp vanilla extract split lengthwise and inside scraped out

½-1 tsp vanilla liquid stevia

2 cups ice

Optional topping: whipped cream chocolate shavings

¼ tsp xanthan gum optional to thicken

DIRECTIONS:

01. Place all ingredients together except ice.

02. Blend on high for just a few seconds to combine.

03. Add ice and blend again for a just a minute to crush ice.

04. Taste and adjust stevia if needed.

05. Serves 4 at about 1 1/2 cups each or serve 2 for a larger portion!

06. Recipe Notes

07. If after you blend, it's not thick enough to your liking, try adding 1/4 -1/2 tsp xanthan gum to thicken.

NUTRITION:

Calories 217

Calories from Fat 207

Total Fat 23 g

Saturated Fat 13 g

Cholesterol 81 mg

Sodium 22 mg

Potassium 44 mg

Total Carbohydrates 2 g

Protein 1 g

KETO CHEESECAKE

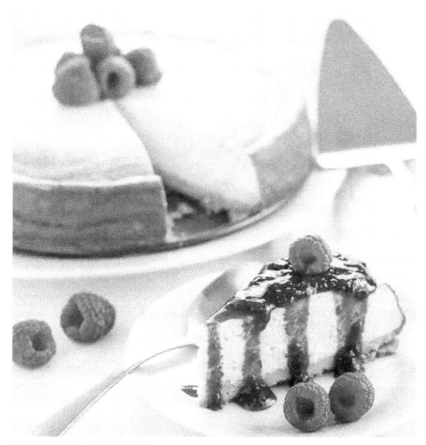

SERVING: 16 SLICES

INGREDIENTS:

Almond Flour Cheesecake Crust

2 cups Blanched almond flour

⅓ cup Butter (measured solid, then melted)

3 Tbsp Erythritol (granular or powdered works fine)

1 tsp Vanilla extract

Keto Cheesecake Filling

32 oz Cream cheese (softened)

1 ¼ cup Powdered erythritol (erythritol must be powdered; can also use powdered monk fruit

sweetener)

3 large Egg

1 Tbsp Lemon juice

1 tsp Vanilla extract

DIRECTIONS:

01. Preheat the oven to 350 degrees F (177 degrees C). Grease a 9 in (23 cm) spring form pan (or you can line the bottom with parchment paper).

02. To make the almond flour cheesecake crust, stir the almond flour, melted butter, erythritol, and vanilla extract in a medium bowl, until well combined. The dough will be slightly crumbly. Press the dough into the bottom of the prepared pan. Bake for about 10-12 minutes, until barely golden. Let cool at least 10 minutes.

03. Meanwhile, beat the cream cheese and powdered sweetener together at low to medium speed until fluffy. Beat in the eggs, one at a time. Finally, beat in the lemon juice and vanilla extract. (Keep the mixer at low to medium the whole time; too high speed will introduce too many air bubbles, which we don't want.)

04. Pour the filling into the pan over the crust. Smooth the top with a spatula (use a pastry spatula for a smoother top if you have one).

05. Bake for about 45-55 minutes, until the center is almost set, but still jiggly.

06. Remove the cheesecake from the oven. If the edges are stuck to the pan, run a knife around the edge (don't remove the spring form edge yet). Cool in the pan on the counter to room temperature, then refrigerate for at least 4 hours (preferably overnight), until completely set. (Do not try to remove the cake from the pan before chilling.)

07. Serve with fresh raspberry sauce if desired.

NUTRITION:

Calories 325

Fat 31 g

Protein 7 g

Total Carbs 6 g

Net Carbs 5 g

Fiber 1 g

Sugar 2 g

KETO RASPBERRY FAT BOMBS

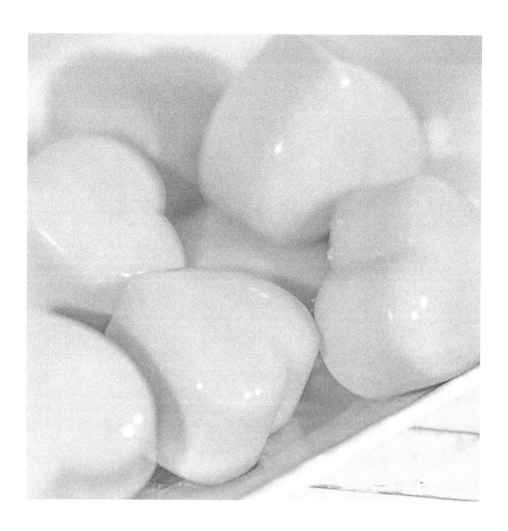

INGREDIENTS:

1 pk Raspberry Sugar Free Jello 9g packet

15 g Gelatin Powder

½ cup water boiling

½ cup Heavy Cream

DIRECTIONS:

01. Dissolve gelatin and jello in boiling water.

02. Add the cream slowly while stirring and continue to stir for 1 minute. If you add the cold cream in all at once and don't thoroughly mix, the jellies will split creating a

layered effect.

03. Pour the mixture into candy molds and set in the fridge for at least 30 minutes. Enjoy!

NUTRITION:

Calories 21 kcal

Carbohydrates 0.1 g

Protein 0.4 g

Fat 2 g

Saturated Fat 1 g

Polyunsaturated Fat 0.1 g

Monounsaturated Fat 0.5 g

Cholesterol 6 mg

Sodium 3 mg

Potassium 4 mg

Sugar 0.005 g

KETO MUG CAKE

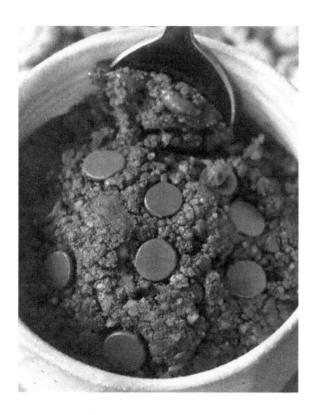

INGREDIENTS:

⅓ cup almonds or pecans, or 6 Tbsp almond flour

1 Tbsp + 2 tsp cocoa powder

1 Tbsp sugar or sweetener of choice pinch stevia, or additional 2 tsp sugar

⅛ Tsp salt

¼ tsp baking powder

3 Tbsp milk of choice (or 2 if using liquid sweetener)

¼ tsp pure vanilla extract

Optional, chocolate chips or sugar free chocolate chips

DIRECTIONS:

01. Combine all ingredients in a greased ramekin or small mug.

02. Either bake in a preheated 350F oven for about 10 minutes, or cook in the microwave. If microwaving, time will vary depending on wattage and desired gooeyness. I started with 30 seconds, then added two 15-second intervals after that.

03. The cake will look a bit gooey when it comes out, and it firms up as it cools. But there's no need to wait for it to firm up too much — this cake is meant to be eaten straight from the mug!

NUTRITION:

Calories 195

Total fat 16.6 g

Cholesterol 0 mg

Sodium 292 mg

Total Carbohydrate 9.8 g

Protein 7.7 g

STRAWBERRY-FILLED FAT BOMBS

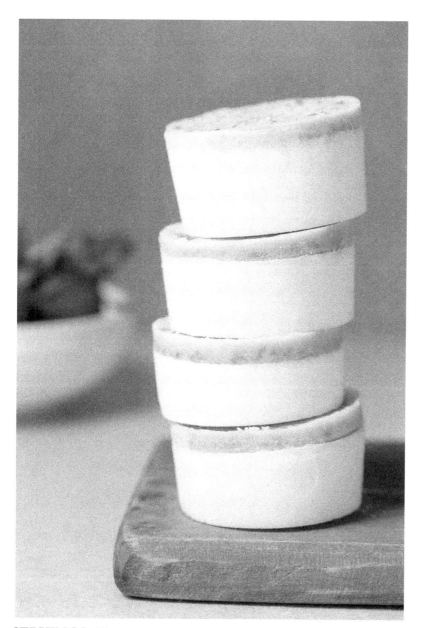

SERVINGS: 15

INGREDIENTS:

⅓ cup coconut butter

⅓ cup coconut oil + 1 Tbsp

½ Tbsp cocoa powder

8-10 drops of liquid stevia to taste

⅓ cup fresh strawberries, diced (about 75g)

1 Tbsp unsweetened shredded coconut

DIRECTIONS:

01. In a bain-marie, add the coconut butter, 1/3 cup coconut oil, cocoa powder and a few drops of liquid stevia. Heat until fully melted.

02. Meanwhile, in a small frying pan, add the fresh strawberries and a few spoonfuls of water. Cook over medium heat until soft. Mash with a fork. Add the berries to a blender with 1 Tbsp of melted coconut oil and a few more drops of liquid stevia. Blend until smooth.

03. Fill molds with the melted coconut mixture. Add about 1 tsp of the strawberry mixture into each mold. Sprinkle with a few shreds of unsweetened coconut.

04. Place in the fridge until fully hardened; at least a couple of hours or overnight. Pop out of the molds and store in an air-tight container in the fridge.

05. Enjoy!

NUTRITION:

Per Fat Bomb

Calories 106

Carbs 2 g

Fibber 1 g

Net Carbs 1 g

Fat 11 g

Protein 1 g

Sugar 1 g

BACON WRAPPED CHEESE STICKS

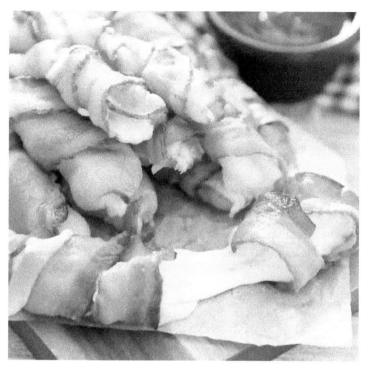

SERVINGS: 12

INGREDIENTS:

12 string cheese or mozzarella cheese sticks

36 strips pre-cooked packaged bacon

DIRECTIONS:

01. Preheat oven to 425°F. Line a large baking sheet with foil or parchment paper.

02. Starting at one end of a cheese stick, carefully wrap one strip of bacon around it, overlapping bacon halfway each time to help secure the bacon in place.

Because the bacon is pre-cooked it will be a little harder to wrap, but the light pink and fat portions should still be pretty flexible. When you reach the end of your bacon, tuck the end into one of the folds to keep it from unwrapping. Repeat with 1-2 more strips of bacon until your cheese is completely covered, including ends of cheese.

03. Place finished wrapped cheese stick on a baking sheet. Repeat with remaining

cheese and bacon. Bake in the oven for about 6-10 minutes, or until bacon is crisp and before cheese completely loses its form.

NUTRITION:

Amount Per Serving (1 biscuit)

Calories 258

Calories from Fat 144

Total Fat 16 g

Saturated Fat 10 g

Cholesterol 45 mg

Sodium 215 mg

Potassium 198 mg

Total Carbohydrates 21 g

Sugars 1 g

Protein 6g

LOADED CAULIFLOWER

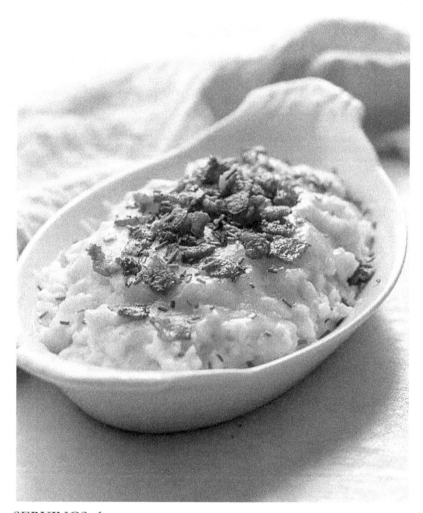

SERVINGS: 6

INGREDIENTS:

1 lb cauliflower florettes

4 oz sour cream

1 cup grated cheddar cheese

2 slices cooked bacon crumbled

2 Tbsp snipped chives

3 Tbsp butter

¼ tsp garlic powder

Salt and pepper to taste

DIRECTIONS:

01. Cut the cauliflower into florettes and add them to a microwave safe bowl. Add 2 tablespoons of water and cover with cling film. Microwave for 5-8 minutes, depending on your microwave, until completely cooked and tender. Drain the excess water and let sit uncovered for a minute or two. (Alternately, steam your cauliflower the conventional way. You may need to squeeze a little water out of the cauliflower after cooking.)

02. Add the cauliflower to a food processor and process until fluffy. Add the butter, garlic powder, and sour cream and process until it resembles the consistency of mashes potatoes. Remove the mashed cauliflower to a bowl and add most of the chives, saving some to add to the top later. Add half of the cheddar cheese and mix by hand. Season with salt and pepper.

03. Top the loaded cauliflower with the remaining cheese, remaining chives and bacon. Put back into the microwave to melt the cheese or place the cauliflower under the broiler for a few minutes.

04. I visually divide the cauliflower into sixths. Serving size is approximately 1/3-1/2 cup.

NUTRITION:

Calories 199 kcal

Carbohydrates 5 g

Protein 8 g

Fat 17 g

Saturated Fat 10 g

Polyunsaturated Fat 1 g

Monounsaturated Fat 5 g

Cholesterol 46 mg

Sodium 242 mg

Potassium 291 mg

Fiber 2 g

BROCCOLI SALAD

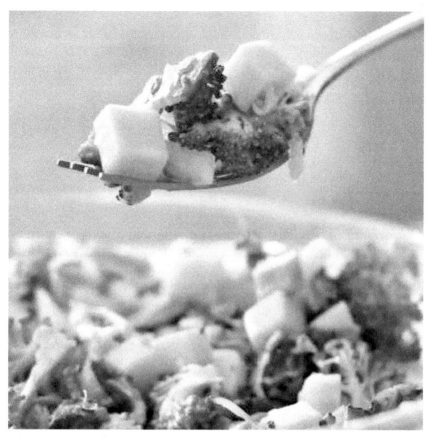

SERVING SIZE: 1 CUP

YIELD: 10

INGREDIENTS:

Dressing:

1 cup mayonnaise

2 Tbsp apple cider vinegar

¼ cup sugar (or equivalent sweetener of your choice)

For the Broccoli Salad

4 cups Broccoli cut into bite-sized pieces, stalk and all(except tough parts)

5 strips cooked bacon

½ cup onion, finely diced (I use white onion)

1 cup dried Cranberries

1 cup cheddar cheese (cut into ¼ inch cubes)

⅛ cup sunflower seeds

⅛ cup pumpkin seeds

DIRECTIONS:

01. For the Dressing:

02. Whisk together the dressing ingredients and adjust them to your personal taste. Set aside.

03. For the Broccoli Salad:

04. Set a skillet to medium heat. Lay the bacon strips in and cook covered until browned. Turn

the bacon over and cook covered a few more minutes until browned but NOT burned.

05. Remove bacon to a cutting board and chop when cool to touch into 1/4 inch pieces. Set aside.

06. Meanwhile chop and measure broccoli, onion and cheese and pour into a large bowl.

07. Add the chopped bacon and remaining ingredients.

08. Pour the dressing over the assembled salad ingredients and stir gently until all parts of the salad are evenly coated.

09. Serve at room temperature of chilled. This salad can be made a day ahead and refrigerated. It holds up to a week in the fridge covered as leftovers.

NUTRITION:

Calories 355

Total Fat 25 g

Saturated Fat 6 g

Trans Fat 0 g

Unsaturated Fat 18 g

Cholesterol 28 mg

Sodium 476 mg

Carbohydrates 28 g

Fiber 4 g

Sugar 19 g

Protein 8 g

PEANUT BUTTER PUDDING

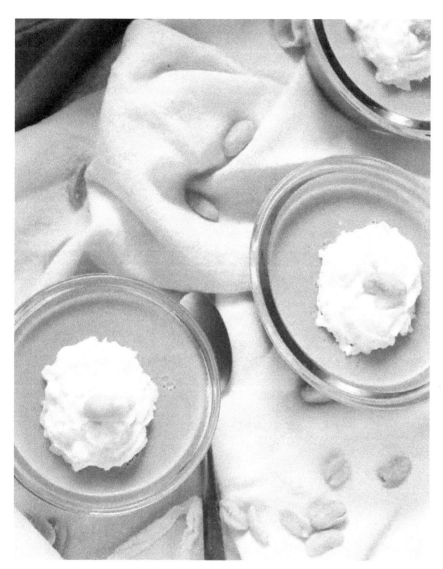

SERVINGS: 4

INGREDIENTS:

2 cups Unsweetened Cashew Milk

¼ cup Natural Peanut Butter no sugar added

¼ cup Gentle Sweet

2 tsp Vanilla

½ cup Water

1 Tbsp Just Gelatin

DIRECTIONS:

01. In a medium saucepan, combine unsweetened cashew milk, natural peanut butter, Gentle Sweet, and vanilla.

02. Heat over medium heat until peanut butter has melted and mixture is smooth.

03. In a small bowl, sprinkle 1 Tablespoon Just Gelatin over 1/2 cup cool water.

04. Let sit for about 30 seconds or so, then stir well.

05. Add gelatin mixture to pudding and stir well.

06. Pour into 4 ramekins and refrigerate for at least 2 hours before serving.

NUTRITION:

Calories 140

Fat 9.5

Carbs 12.5

Sugar Alcohols 9

Fiber 1

Net Carbs 2.5

Protein 6

PEANUT BUTTER MUG CAKE

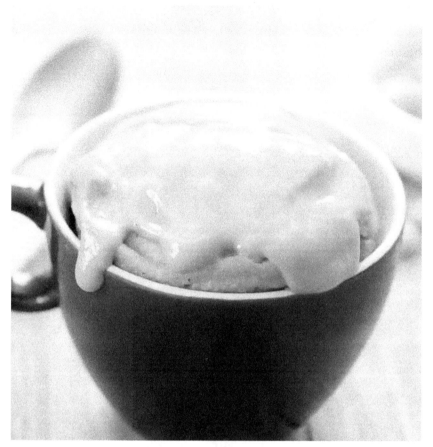

A single serving microwave peanut butter mug cake that is only three ingredients. It's quick, easy and is also keto-friendly, low carb, wheat flour free, and gluten free.

INGREDIENTS:

2 ½ Tbsp natural creamy unsalted peanut butter

2 ½ tsp Natural Mate All Purpose Granular Stevia or sugar substitute of your choice equivalent to 1 Tbsp + 2 tsp sugar

1 large egg

DIRECTIONS:

01. In a microwave-safe mug that can hold at least 12 oz of liquid, add all ingredients. Mix with a whisk until batter is completely smooth and egg is fully incorporated with

no egg streaks remaining. Your batter should look like melted peanut butter.

02. Cook in the microwave at full power for about 1 minute. I used a 1000 watt microwave.

You may need to adjust cooking time and power if your microwave is a different wattage. Cake is best enjoyed warm.

NUTRITION:

Calories 318

Calories from Fat 225

Total Fat 25 g

Saturated Fat 4 g

Cholesterol 210 mg

Sodium 80 mg

Potassium 337 mg

Total Carbohydrates 9 g

Dietary Fiber 3 g

Sugars 1 g

Protein 15 g

CPSIA information can be obtained
at www.ICGtesting.com
Printed in the USA
BVHW011408100321
602204BV00008B/318